Biomedical Devices and Sensors

First published 2024 in Great Britain and the United States by ISTE Ltd and John Wiley & Sons, Inc.

ISTE Ltd
27-37 St George's Road
London SW19 4EU
UK

www.iste.co.uk

John Wiley & Sons, Inc.
111 River Street
Hoboken, NJ 07030
USA

www.wiley.com

Library of Congress Control Number: 2024936647

British Library Cataloguing-in-Publication Data
A CIP record for this book is available from the British Library
ISBN 978-1-78630-946-4

Contents

Foreword

Medical devices have a long history. It was in Egypt that the first traces of prostheses and orthoses were found. These major discoveries highlight the Egyptians' mastery of textile manufacturing techniques, metallurgy and woodworking. These discoveries also show their medical knowledge, as well as their understanding of anatomical, morphological and aesthetic issues, the latter two being essential to help with the treatment.

The treatises by Galen and Amboise Paré demonstrate the constant progress of medical devices over the centuries, mainly concerning the development of war medicine.

It was especially from the 19th century, following on from the Industrial Revolution, that their development accelerated. The first implantable hip was invented in the late 19th century, and the first textile-based cardiovascular implants were created in the 1950s, as was the first pacemaker.

Medical devices are now fully fledged means of treatment and diagnosis. They are used in many pathological situations. Among them, there are products as varied as surgical masks, glasses, compression stockings, lumbar belts, orthopedic implants, X-ray machines, blood glucose measuring devices and, more recently, smartphone applications allowing for a more precise support of the patient in their daily life.

Scientific progress, in a more detailed understanding of pathologies, but also progress in engineering sciences such as materials, mechanics, electronics, numerical modeling and artificial intelligence, has made it possible to bring more complex and innovative medical devices to the market.

We are entering a new era in the 21st century. The growth of the population, which is expected to reach 10 billion by the end of the 21st century, its unprecedented ageing, and its growing sedentarization are all factors leading to an increase in chronic pathologies (diabetes, cardiovascular problems, musculoskeletal disorders, etc.) for which medical devices are the treatments of choice.

The availability of medical devices for healthcare professionals and patients has become an important issue. The increasing complexity of the products means that their components are produced and assembled in various locations across the world. Any geopolitical issues can have a direct impact on their availability and quality.

The processes for marketing authorization as well as for reimbursements have also been strengthened, as has the case for medicines. Marketing authorizations (CE marking in Europe, FDA approval in the United States, CFDA approvals in China, etc.), and even more so the conditions of access to reimbursement, differ between each major region of the world, and usually between each state. Often based on the compliance of medical devices with technical guidelines or standards, the marketing authorization and reimbursement require more and more. Due to the increasing complexity of the products, they use clinical trials in order to demonstrate their therapeutic efficacy.

The unique nature of medical devices makes it difficult to use the same clinical trial methodologies as for medicines. A placebo for a medical device is often impossible. This peculiarity means that different clinical trial techniques are used, and more recently the use of numerical models, or sensors, has emerged.

In this book, Professor Jérôme Molimard offers an extraordinary perspective on medical devices from their design to their launch on the market. The author describes in detail aspects that are very rarely addressed at the same time. This pedagogical approach first addresses the elements necessary for the implementation of the market, the conformity of which must be demonstrated from the design stage. The use of sensors and numerical models is then described in detail. These two types of tools are essential for the R&D phases, allowing considerable savings in terms of time to bring products to market. In the final part, the book discusses in more detail the methods used in clinical research and biostatistics necessary to demonstrate the efficacy of medical devices.

I am sure this book will be of interest to all students, engineers, health professionals and scientists wishing to better understand medical devices. It is a reference work for understanding their different aspects.

Reynald CONVERT
Technology and Intelligence Director
Thuasne
France

1

Medical Device: Definition, History and Economic Background

1.1. Definition

Everyday life in hospitals can provide as many examples of medical devices as necessary to convince someone of the diversity and the significant importance of this sector in modern medicine: hip prostheses, insulin pumps, pacemakers, magnetic resonance imaging (MRI) devices, as well as syringes, crutches, wheelchairs or dressings. Despite their diversity, they all belong to the category of medical devices. A definition can be extracted from the Regulation (EU) 2017/745 of the European Parliament and of the Council of April 5, 2017.

> *"Medical device" means any instrument, apparatus, appliance, software, implant, reagent, material or other article intended by the manufacturer to be used, alone or in combination, for human beings for one or more of the following specific medical purposes:*
>
> *– diagnosis, prevention, monitoring, prediction, prognosis, treatment or alleviation of disease;*

> *– diagnosis, monitoring, treatment and alleviation of, or compensation for, an injury or disability;*
>
> *– investigation, replacement or modification of the anatomy or of a physiological or pathological process or state;*
>
> *– providing information by means of in vitro examination of specimens derived from the human body, including organ, blood and tissue donations, and which does not achieve its principal intended action by pharmacological, immunological or metabolic means, in or on the human body, but which may be assisted in its function by such means.*
>
> *The following products shall also be deemed to be medical devices:*
>
> *– devices for the control or support of conception;*
>
> *– products specifically intended for the cleaning, disinfection or sterilization of devices as referred to in Article 1(4) and in the first paragraph of this chapter.*

As can be seen, the category of medical device is defined by its claim (human care, in a medical meaning) and by the means used (all means except pharmacological). It is interesting to see that software is mentioned in this definition, and thus, a piece of software that influences the medical process in some way is considered a medical device.

There is indeed a gray area between medical devices and other common devices. In this gray area lie most of the healthcare Internet of Things (IoT) gadgets or smartphone applications (e.g. cardiac monitoring, physical activity monitoring and brain sensing headbands). Most of these are *not* registered as medical devices and pretend to be sports or well-being applications, even if they target those who are anxious about their health and may suffer from chronic diseases. The quality of such measurement and/or processing, their influence on the customer's health and the use of such amounts of personal data both by medical professionals or even private companies must be put into question by regulatory authorities as well as by the consumer themselves.

1.2. Examples of medical devices

The history of medical devices is directly related to that of techniques. It borrows from mechanics, optics, electronics and computer sciences and applies these to medicine. Surgeons in the Neolithic period performed brain surgery; copper dilators for urethral stenosis from the ancient Egyptians have been found; we could also refer to Mayan glasses. Should all of these be considered medical devices?

1.2.1. *Surgery equipment*

Audry and Ghislain (2009) consider that the history of modern medical devices begins in 1894 with E. Fournier, who commercialized the first syringe presenting industrial features, normalization and large diffusion. A few years later, in 1904, the "Dräger-Roth" inhalator, set-up in Germany, opened the way to modern anesthesia.

The hip prosthesis is a good example of advances in materials and material processing in a health application. At the beginning of the 20th century, surgeons tried to insert materials into the body to replace lost cartilage. But this created bio-compatibility or structure mechanics problems. The solution was found in the UK: totally replacing the joint. After an attempt with ivory, the first functional prosthesis using Chromium-Cobalt-Molybdenum alloy was proposed in 1936 by Dr. Bohlman, but there was a high friction coefficient, with a lot of wear particles diffused in the body. Polytetrafluoroethylene (PTFE) appeared in 1959 and in the 1970s Prof. Boutin proposed a total hip replacement with a ceramic head. In the same period, Prof. G. Bousquet improved mobility by adding a second degree of freedom to hip prosthesis with the concept of double mobility prosthesis, reducing the risk of dislocation.

The fight against strokes was one of the biggest adventures for humans in the second half of the 20th century and medical devices were the weapons of cardiac surgeons forged by engineers. In 1950, J. Hoops developed the first prototype of the pacemaker. This model was cumbersome and not easy to live with because it was external and required a power supply. The first internal pacemaker was developed and implanted a few years later, in 1958, by Drs. R. Elmqvist and A. Senning in Sweden. In fact, during the 1950s, many independent projects came out in Europe and North America.

This period saw many advances in bio-materials, and some of these resulted in important applications in cardiology. For example, Prof. A. Carpentier developed the first bio-prosthesis: the human mitral valve was replaced by a bio-prosthesis based on a valve from a pig. The original system wore off after few years; now, the third generation lifespan is 25 years. During the 1970s and the 1980s, electronic engineering allowed for the miniaturization of all of the systems. In 2008, after many years of research, Carpentier started the Carmat company, which developed a totally artificial heart, taking advantage of the previous developments in cardiac regulation for pacemakers, but also bio-materials, in particular animal-based materials. The first implantation of a totally artificial heart succeeded in 2013.

Miniaturization of medical devices totally changed the way in which surgeons practiced operations. In 1973, Profs. Bruhat and Manhes achieved the first endoscopic surgery of an extra-uterine pregnancy in Clermont-Ferrand (France). Since then, the advances in microelectronics, medical imaging and augmented reality have made endoscopic surgery possible in many fields: general surgery, urology or even cardiac surgery, with endoscopic placement of stents or cardiac valves. This new paradigm in surgery strongly decreases the invasiveness of surgery and thus increases the chance of the patient's recovery, limits the side effects of the surgery and finally decreases the overall medical cost.

Finally, insulin pumps are another interesting example of a medical device, which have become the gold standard for chronic diseases. The innovation came from Germany, with glycemia measurement units proposed in 1969, and 10 years later, we saw the first pump. The technical problem that lay behind this is the insulin regulation that controls the patient's diabetes. Now, both the measurement unit and pump are miniaturized enough to be implanted into the human body. The last step is to connect the measurement to the pump controller, but this raises more than just technical questions: what would happen in the case of a problem? Who is ultimately responsible for the care?

1.2.2. *Medical imaging*

Perhaps the biggest change in medical practices over the 50 past years is medical imaging.

W. Röntgen discovered X-ray radiations in 1895 in Germany. Although he was following some pioneers' works, he was the first to publish material on it. He discovered that X-rays pass through solids. After making an image of a woman's hand, he understood the great interest of X-rays in medicine. The technique spread very quickly: the first surgery under X-rays was performed by J. Hall-Edwards only 1 year later in the UK, and in 1896 a Georgian physician I. Tarkhanishvili discovered that X-rays affect metabolism. Soon after, side effects were reported: hair loss, burns, etc. An early researcher developed a type of cancer due to the radiation produced by X-rays and died in 1904. Advances in X-ray generation and detection saw a perambulation in the history of modern physics, with names such as M. von Laue, W.L. Bragg or W.E. Bragg. We ended up with W. Coolidge who invented X-ray tubes with a continuous emission in 1913 and M. Skłodowska-Curie, who, in 1914, developed mobile radiography units for soldiers in World War I (Figure 1.1). Medical imaging using X-rays is based on the absorption properties of high atomic numbers such as calcium, which provokes a contrast. Bone or dental imaging is straightforward; what is more, after calibration, the bone density can be directly deduced from image intensity maps. Cardiovascular imaging is possible using contrast agents. In this 2D projection form, X-rays are used for dental applications, detection of skeleton problems, but also in the diagnosis of various diseases (pneumonia, lung cancer, pulmonary edema, bowel obstruction, gallstones, kidney stones, etc.), or for implant follow-ups. One image only is a conical projection; by taking various images at different points of view, it is possible to back-project the X-rays (Radon transform) and to reconstruct the whole volume. Of course, the cost for that is higher irradiation and some very recent advances could reduce this irradiation level. In 1968, G. Charpak developed a new detector in France, the "multi-wire detection chamber" that divides the irradiation received by the patient by a factor of ten. In 2008, this detector was implanted by EOS Imaging (Paris, France) in an integrated X-rays system that reconstructs 3D images by using two images of the patient and a knowledge basis.

Compared to X-rays, MRI is a relatively new technology that first began in 1946 with the discovery of the magnetic resonance phenomenon independently by F. Bloch and E. Purcell (USA). Magnetic resonance is a physical phenomenon that occurs on atoms when they are subjected to a high magnetic field: they reorient and relax into their original position if the magnetic field stops, emitting radio signals. MRI imaging is based on the different relaxation times (named T1, T2). It was used first for chemical and physical analysis, and only in 1971 was it used for medical applications by R. Damadian, P. Lauterbur and P. Mansfield. It was necessary to speed-up the mathematical processing to make it useful in medicine. Then, studying different kinds of tissues outlined differences, specifically for cancerous tissues. As already introduced for X-ray imaging, MRI took advantage of multiple image exposure to perform 3D reconstructions. Developments in MRI are strongly related to the generation of magnetic fields. With the progress of superconductors, MRI systems have increased the magnetic field from 0.5 T to 1.5 T or 3.0 T which is common in clinical practice nowadays, and up to 7 T for research applications[1]. Besides this orientation, which uses more power and more expensive equipment, other orientations consist of decreasing the magnetic field by the optimization of the signal-to-noise ratio with numerical processing and MRI sequence optimization. The MRI sequence can enhance tissue visibility and MRI suppliers compete for the quality of the sequences they propose. The last major innovation – but again in the engineering field rather than in the scientific one – in 1996, Fonar (New York, USA) proposed an open MRI where the patient is not in a supine position but in a standing one. This gives better representativity and comfort for the patient and opens the way to functional MRI with patients in movement. Innovations, still in the research field, are now being driven by molecules heavier than water, that can give information on the biochemical state of the patient, for example, their inflammation level.

1 Note that such an electromagnetic field constrains what is inside the field to strictly nonmagnetic materials.

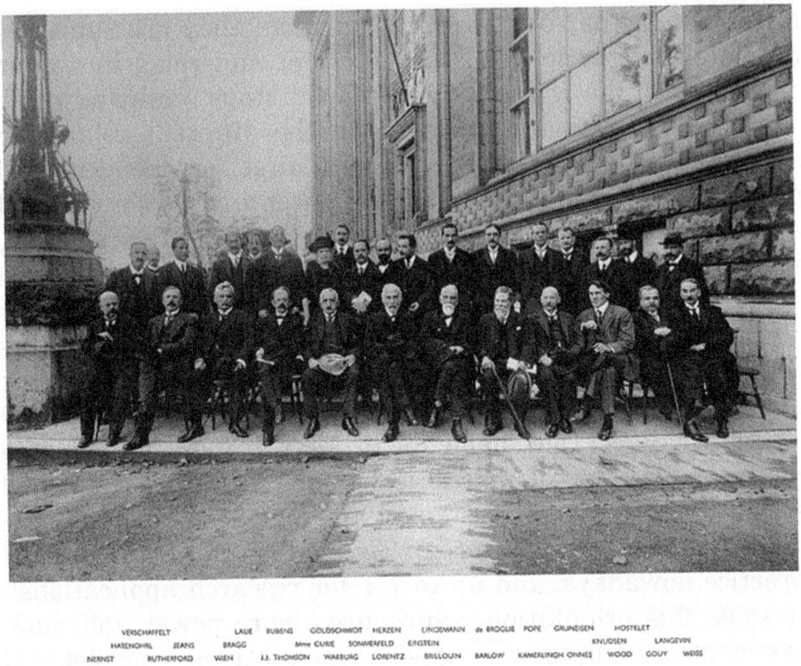

Figure 1.1. *Photograph of the second Solvay conference. Among the participants, W.L. Bragg, M. Curie and M. von Laue (public domain)*

Along with MRI, computer tomography (CT) scans are expensive techniques whose effects on the body are questionable. The last system presented here – even if this short-list is still somewhat incomplete – is ultrasound imaging. L. Spallanzani in Italy discovered that bats were using sounds he could not hear to orient themselves (echolocation) and he was the first to describe these sounds from 1000 to 200,000 Hz. Thanks to P. Langevin (France), humans have been able to reproduce what bats can do since 1915: he invented a device that could detect objects at the bottom of the sea, the hydrophone. This is considered to be the “first transducer”. The real history of ultrasound imaging began in 1942 in Austria: K. Dussik transmitted an ultrasound beam through the human skull to detect brain tumors. The piezoelectric crystal (PZT) first emits ultrasound and then receives the echo. The first equipment came out in 1948 to detect gallstones (G.D. Ludwig, USA). It was a simple unidirectional system (A-mode ultrasound), but very soon (1949–1951) D. Howry and J. Holmes (USA) pioneered 2D imaging, known as B-mode ultrasound equipment. The most well-known applications are in obstetrics and the detection of tumors – in particular breast tumors, and those in pneumology or urology. In 1966, pulse-Doppler ultrasound imaging came out (D. Baker, D. Watkins and J. Reid) leading to blood flow imaging and angiology applications. Applications of ultrasounds concern any soft tissue that can transmit a mechanical vibration. The idea of coupling medical imaging and mechanical loading came out in 1991 thanks to J. Ophir (USA). A simple analysis shows that such a technique gives an image of the tissue elasticity, and due to this, it has been called elastography. The principal characteristic of ultrasound elastography – compared to MRI – is that the transducer itself can generate the load. In 2004 J.L. Genisson (France) proposed the ultrasonic shear wave elastography that could propagate a wave inside the body. Because it enhances the differences in tissue stiffness, elastography is more efficient in the detection of tumors than the classical B-mode. Now, modern ultrasound systems have a frequency range from 1 to 18 MHz depending on the penetration sought (acoustic absorption varies with the square of the frequency) and a sensor arrangement gathers 128–960 transducers, even 3,000 in specific cases.

Now, ultrasound techniques are developing in a very novel direction. Because ultrasounds are transmitting energy, it is possible to increase and to concentrate this energy in small areas, provoking local heat, and as a consequence cell apoptosis. This new technique, known as high-intensity focused ultrasound (HIFU), is therefore a local noninvasive ablation technique. It can be easily image guided by decreasing the power. HIFU was ideated in the 1950s by W. Fry and F. Fry in Cincinnati (USA), but the first medical developments came out in Europe. In 2006, F. Murat

(France) demonstrated its efficiency on prostate cancer, and this approach has been approved by the EU.

1.3. Medical device industry

1.3.1. *The industrial sector*

The sector of medical devices is one which is not very old. One of the main characteristics of this sector is the diversity of the actors: physicians, engineers, pharmacologists, lawyers, etc. This diversity is also valid inside each profession; among physicians for example, medical device innovation may come from cardiologists, physical medicine or orthopedists. Of course, this is the same for engineers, with biomechanics, electronics, automation or artificial intelligence. Teams that contain an entrepreneur, an engineer and a physician will always be a boost to success for any start-up project.

The youth of the sector, and the dynamism of the actors of the medical field, explains that 95%[2] of the activity is performed by small- (B Braun, Carmat, Supersonic Imaging, EOS Imaging, etc.) and medium-sized companies (Thuasne, Sigvaris, Ossür, L&R, etc.). Of course, some of the classical optics companies are present (Philips, Zeiss, Seimens, etc.). Even some pure players are big enough to count as multinationals (Abbott, Medtronics, etc.). Now, the European Union wants fewer bigger-sized companies.

Because of this dispersion of the players, quantification cannot be accurate, but it is admitted that the medical

---

2 Economic figures for this paragraph come from the following:
MedTechEurope (2002). MedTech Europe's facts & figures 2022 [Online]. Available at: https://www.medtecheurope.org/resource-library/medtech-europes-facts-and-figures-2022/.
EFPIA (2002). The pharmaceutical industry in figures – Key data [Online]. Available at: https://www.efpia.eu/media/637143/the-pharmaceutical-industry-in-figures-2022.pdf.
PIPAME Report (2011).

devices represent one-third of the pharmacological market (187 €bn in 2005). The medical device market has a 4.8% growth each year, whereas the pharmacological market growth is 5.8% (EU) or 5.6% (USA). Another important difference is the lifecycle of the products: all of the regulation processes for medical devices is copy-pasted from drugs, but the development lasts for 5–6 years, whereas that of drugs is around 12 years. The time on the market for a medical device is also half of that of a drug (5 years instead of 8 years).

The U.S. market is the largest, with 239 €bn (~43.5%); the European market represents 150 €bn (27.3%) followed by Asia (with China, 7.2%). Following this trend, the United States is the major supplier, followed by the European Union. Within Europe, Germany covers 31% of European production, France 16%, followed by the UK and Italy (11% each).

1.3.2. *Importance of medical device in the economy*

One way to qualify the importance of the medical device industry in the economy should be to look at its growth potential: in France, the growth rate is 4–6% and 50 companies are established each year. The number of European patent applications was 15,300 in 2021, with a 0.8% growth compared to the previous year. All of this makes the sector an important source of growth. In comparison, the number of patents in the pharmaceutical industry remains stable with 9,000 applications in 2021. The medical device industry employed 800,000 people in Europe (PIPAME Report 2011), most of them in Germany, then Italy, UK and France. The pharmaceutical industry represents 840,000 employees at the same moment. This industry represents 0.8% of European production and 0.3% of employment.

The weight of medical devices in health expenses is close to 6% (5.2% in the United States and 7.6% in the European Union). The rough expense per capita in the European Union is close to 295€ and can be estimated as 635€ in the United States. The investment in research and development in the United States is close to 11%, whereas the mean ratio is 8% in Europe, with countries such as Germany, Sweden or Switzerland being close to the value of the United States. As a comparison, the pharmaceutical industry inversion in R&D is 16%.

PERSONAL PRACTICE.– Find the key data for your own country. What are the main actors in the field?

2

Medical Device Design and Development

2.1. Medical device design is much more than device design

Medical device designers must pursue two main objectives: adding value to the end user while finding a profitable business model in the context of a highly regulated environment and – sometimes – life-critical applications. In addition, in the past 10 years, the new solution in development must be more efficient and more cost-effective than existing solutions to take advantage of national medical care systems.

As it can be seen, the design of a new medical device is a multi-dimensional problem requiring various skills throughout the process (engineering, healthcare, regulatory affairs, business, social science, etc.). Figure 2.1 gives a rough idea of the design phase in the medical device development flowchart. Even if the regulatory design phase appears late (after the proof of concept testing), the research and development engineers must take into account these requirements earlier in order to minimize the amount of work for medical device compliance. In particular, the "design history file" is a first step in the quality insurance, which is mandatory for Medical Device European or American certification.

Specifically, in medical device design, a multidisciplinary team must work together in alignment with an end user's need. The question of the risk and the quality is central. For example, a pacemaker has a very high required reliability, considering that a failure would almost instantaneously lead to the patient's death. However, medical devices are not always as critical; the risk associated with a surgical mask is fairly low – even if it has to be carefully addressed anyway. Risk mitigation is therefore one of the most sensitive aspects of medical device development.

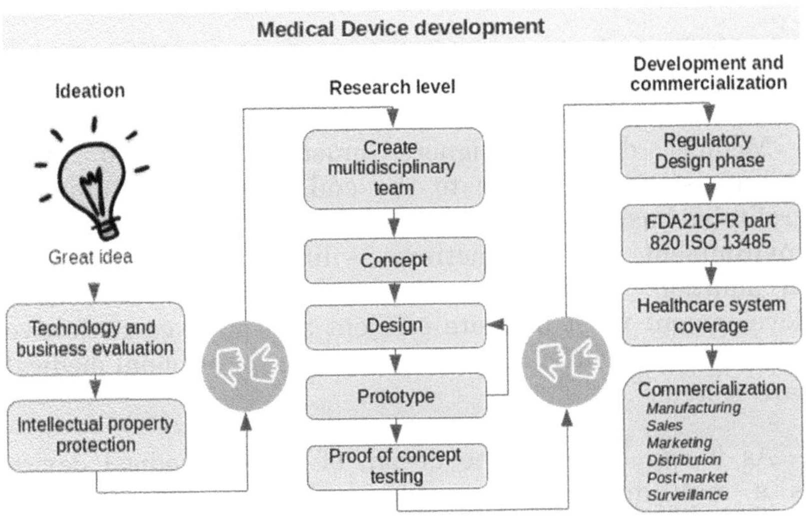

Figure 2.1. *Medical device development (adapted from E-infochip 2018). For a color version of this figure, see www.iste.co.uk/molimard/biomedicaldevices.zip*

Risk/benefit balance is a central aspect in medical practice and the practitioner is always looking to reduce the patient's risk related to a medical treatment (including risks associated with the medical device) and to maximize the benefit, specifically the medical device efficiency.

2.2. Product ideation and conceptualization

Traditionally, medical device innovation starts with analyzing and identifying the market, the need of which is unmet, or a new, efficient way to address particular needs. These needs could be anything that delivers a solution in monitoring health, enhanced care delivery solutions, devices or technologies to deliver better administration or anything that supports health and human life. Innovation supposes that the way to address these needs is new in some aspects and can give rise to patents.

Product ideation and conceptualization ideally starts with the following:

1) Identification of a need

Uncovered or badly covered needs can arise when speaking with patients or practitioners with open questions. The way to address this need can derive from spontaneous ideation but can also come from techniques such as design thinking. Specifically, to the medical environment, compliance to a treatment (from the patient) and the acceptability of a new idea (from the practitioners or the patient) are as important as technical efficiency. Therefore, design by use is a good strategy. In many cases, commercial failure would be avoided by consulting specialists in the sociology of uses or in intercultural representation.

Time to market has to be limited; besides the necessary design flowchart (development, prototyping, etc.), the success very much depends on the gap between the real need of the market, the comprehension the development team has and its translation into a relevant product definition (desired performances for a specific need).

The United States or European Union classify medical devices into categories corresponding to a certain risk level, as detailed in Table 2.1. For existing devices, the Food and Drugs Administration (FDA) provides an online device database[1,2]. These categories are important because they define the requirement for compliance with local standards.

2) Intellectual property protection

Once you are done with the product definition and idea, you need to look for any pre-existing intellectual property (patents, published research) on the proposed idea or similar; this might actually prevent you from using the technology, or applying a patent to it and convincing investors. Background research, as well as patenting, are specialized jobs that should be carried out by external consulting firms.

3) Research phase

Both the identification of needs and the intellectual property protection result in the definition of functional specifications. The next phase has been labeled as a reference to a "Research and Development" service that should develop a new medical device. "Research" here could also say risky task, as technical solutions are still poorly known. The research phase will have to include designing a first prototype, testing it both for verification (of specifications) and validation (on how to cover needs). The research phase leads, after iterations on the previous points, to a proof of concept. The body of this chapter aims at giving key information to go through this phase.

1 Available at: https://www.accessdata.fda.gov/scripts/cdrh/cfdocs/cfpcd/classification.cfm.

2 For European rules, see: https://health.ec.europa.eu/system/files/2021-10/mdcg_2021-24_en_0.pdf.

	USA	EU
Class I	Example: stethoscopes, bandages and medical gloves. – Low-risk devices that are relatively simple in design. – Self-register product with the FDA. – QMS normally complies with CFR part 820: general control, though some devices are exempt.	Example: wheelchair, stethoscopes and spectacles. – Low-risk devices. – Self-assessment.
Class II	Example: ultrasonic diagnostic equipment, X-rays and needles. – Medium risk devices that are more complex in design. – 510(k) pre-market approval process is required for most. – QMS must comply with CFR part 820: general control and special controls (design controls).	Example: Class IIa: dental fillings, surgical clamps and tracheotomy tubes. Class IIb: condoms, lung ventilators and bone fixation plates. – Medium-risk devices. – Notified body approval required.
Class III	Example: balloon catheters, pacemakers and heart valves. – High-risk devices. – FDA should inspect facility. – Clinical trials likely. – Malfunction is absolutelssy unacceptable.	Example: pacemakers, heart valves and implanted cerebral simulators. – High-risk devices. – Notified body approval required.

Table 2.1. *Medical device classification. QMS: quality management system; CFR: Code of Federal Regulation*

4) Development and commercialization

A proof of concept must run the gamut of the notified body approval. This step opens the way to industrialization and commercialization. Quality assessment should be the constant preoccupation in the industrialization process (see the ISO 13485 *Medical devices – Quality management systems – Requirements for regulatory purposes*).

DESIGN THINKING.–

Design thinking is an innovation management methodology developed at Stanford University by R. Faste. It comes in different versions, but the most common version has five steps: *understanding*, *defining*, *ideating*, *prototyping* and *testing*.

2.3. Regional and international standard for addressing regulation and compliance need

Medical device standards are helpful and/or mandatory in specifying and evaluating the requirement for design and performance parameters for a biomedical device. Due to the very large variety of devices, systems or software that lie in the medical device regulation framework, rules are put in place on the quality management and risk management. The responsibility is that of the supplier, even if some tasks can be outsourced. Table 2.2 presents principle standards for quality and risk management.

This international global framework can have some local variations that might lead to rejection of the medical device proposal in the given market. Indeed, recently, U.S. regulation has moved closer to the international standards used in Europe. At present, the 14971:2019 is mandatory both for the European Union and U.S. markets. Even though design controls are defined under FDA 21 CFR 820.30, also known as Current Good Manufacturing Practices (CGMPs) in the

United States, recent evolutions have made FDA 221 CFR 820.30 requirements align with ISO 13485. It is worth noting that FDA regulation is mandatory, while ISO is a voluntary standard that generally speaking does not have legal consequences.

IEC60601-111:2015	**Medical electrical equipment – Part 1–11: General requirements for basic safety and essential performance – collateral standard: Requirements for medical electrical equipment and medical electrical systems used in the home healthcare environment**
	IEC 60601-1-11:2015 applies to the basic safety and essential performance of medical electrical equipment and medical electrical systems for use in the home healthcare environment. It applies regardless of whether the medical electrical equipment or medical electrical system is intended for use by a lay operator or by trained healthcare personnel. The home healthcare environment includes the following: – the dwelling place in which a patient lives; – other places where patients are present both indoors and outdoors, excluding professional healthcare facility environments where operators with medical training are continually available when patients are present.
ISO13485:2016	**Medical devices – Quality management systems – Requirements for regulatory purposes**
	ISO 13485:2016 specifies requirements for a quality management system where an organization needs to demonstrate its ability to provide medical devices and related services that consistently meet customer and applicable regulatory requirements. Such organizations can be involved in one or more stages of the lifecycle, including design and development, production, storage and distribution, installation, or servicing of a medical device and design and development or provision of associated activities (e.g. technical support). ISO 13485:2016 can also be used by suppliers or external parties that provide product, including quality management system-related services to such organizations. Requirements of ISO 13485:2016 are applicable to organizations regardless of their size and regardless of their type, except where explicitly stated. Wherever requirements are specified as applying to medical devices, the requirements apply equally to associated services as supplied by the organization.

ISO/TR24971:2020	**Medical devices – Application of risk management to medical devices**
	ISO/TR 24971:2020 provides guidance in addressing specific areas of ISO 14971:2019 when implementing risk management. This guidance is intended to assist manufacturers and other users of the standard to understand the role of international product safety and process standards in risk management, develop the policy for determining the criteria for risk acceptability, incorporate production and post-production feedback loop into risk management, differentiate between "information for safety" and "disclosure of residual risk", and evaluate overall residual risk.

Table 2.2. *Standards for security, quality and risk management in medical devices*

2.4. EU medical device regulation (MDR2017)

In 2017, the EU moved to a new medical device regulation[3] known as MDR2017. The EU medical device regulation is as follows[4]:

– Step 1: Decide the intended use and classification of the planned medical device.

– Step 2: Establish the necessary processes and resources.

– Step 3: Minimize the risks and fulfill the general safety and performance requirements.

– Step 4: Complete the clinical evaluation.

– Step 5: Compile the technical documentation.

– Step 6: Make arrangements for distribution.

– Step 7: Register the device and the manufacturer.

– Step 8: Complete the conformity assessment.

3 Regulation (EU) 2017/745 on medical devices (MDR) and Regulation (EU) 2017/746 on in vitro diagnostic medical devices (IVDR).

4 Available at: http://eumdr.com/.

– Step 9: Complete the final administrative procedures before launch.

– Step 10: Fulfill the ongoing obligations in the post launch phase.

Difficulty arose when manufacturers realized that the regulation was retroactive, and that all devices already on the market had to be validated with MDR2017.

2.5. Design control regulations (for FDA 21CFR820)

Medical device manufacturers need to follow a quality system – and therefore Design Control guidelines – since the regulatory bodies such as the FDA or European Medicines Agency want to ensure that the medical devices are safe (EU) or safe and efficient (USA) for patients before manufacturers start to market the devices. The design control process might avoid 90% of software failures and 44% of voluntary recalls (Liu 2014). It is mandatory for FDA class II and III and some class I medical devices.

A design quality system folder is made up of (1) Design History File, with records describing the history of a finished device, (2) Device Master Record, containing the procedures and specifications of a finished device, and (3) Device History Record, with all the production history of a finished device. The Design Control enters into the quality system with the other subsystems, namely:

– management control;

– production and process control;

– corrective and preventive actions;

– document records and change control;

– material control;

– facility and equipment control.

The design control process is a complete flowchart from the design input to manufacturing processes to the production phase. It may take into account changes in the post-production feedback. Figure 2.2 depicts an FDA design control process. This is an ongoing process to develop a product that is user-oriented. It includes two control loops: design verification and design validation, and opens the way to major changes through reviews, risk analysis or other changes. Design control guidelines cover the entire life of a medical device, starting from design, production, distribution, use, maintenance and obsolescence. Therefore, the success of design control implementation requires the involvement of both technical and non-technical business divisions, for example, research and development, marketing and customer service.

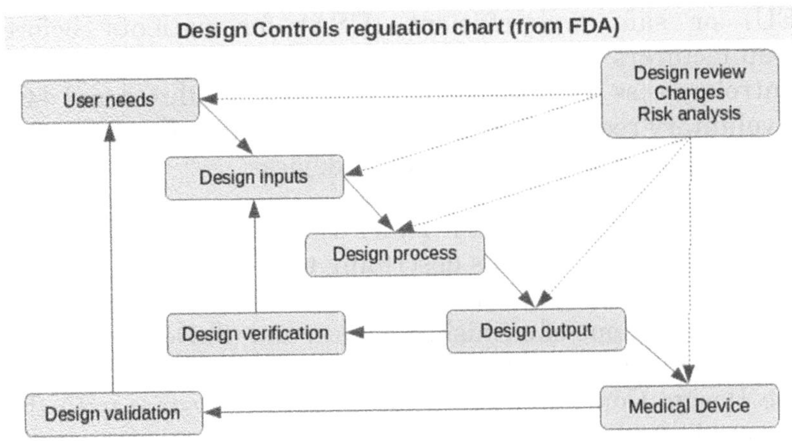

Figure 2.2. *Design control loops according to the FDA (Liu 2014). For a color version of this figure, see www.iste.co.uk/molimard/biomedicaldevices.zip*

The FDA Index for Design Control clause should contain the following: Section A “General”, Section B “Design and development planning”, Section C “Design input”, Section D “Design output”, Section E “Design review”, Section F

"Design verification", Section G "Design Validation", Section H "Design transfer", Section I "Design changes" and Section J "Design History File".

Design control aims at establishing and maintaining procedures to control device design:

– *Design and development planning* describes the design activities, responsibilities and interaction between activities; it includes reviewing and updating the documents.

– *Design inputs* are the physical and performance characteristics of a device that are used as a basis for the device development. Design inputs must be documented and updated throughout the process. Inputs cover the device functions, performance, safety and reliability, but also standards and regulatory requirements, corrective and preventive action (CAPA), human factors, maintenance, environment, etc.

– *Design output* is a list of results of the design at each phase and at the end of the process. It must define relevant outputs, an adequate evaluation and conformance and measurable acceptance criteria. Design outputs are the device specifications that must be verified and validated. They will constitute the basis for the *Device Master Record.* The total finished design consists of the device, its packaging, its labeling and the Device Master Record.

– *Design review* is a systematic, documented and comprehensive examination to evaluate the adequacy of design requirements and the capability of the effective device to meet these requirements and eventual problems. It establishes and maintains a set of procedures. Design review identifies at each stage the representatives of all functions concerned and specialists, as well as individuals without direct responsabilities. The *Design History File* will include document results of the design review, date and individuals performing the review.

– *Design verification* checks that the outputs meet the input requirements by providing objective evidence. Therefore, some quantitative, measurable tests are expected. Design verification will review and approve the *Design History File*. The Design verification test reports will be included in the premarket submission (premarket notification of device presenting equivalence to existing devices 510(k)s, de novos, premarket approval application and investigational device exemption).

– *Design validation* examines through objective testing that the device specifications reach user needs and intended use. This has to be seen under defined operating conditions (normal use or other phases) for the initial production lots. Software validation – along with risk analysis – is possible, when appropriate. Animal studies, cadaveric studies or clinical studies are more frequently used. Design validation activities will be included in the *Design History File*. The design validation results are submitted to the premarket submissions.

– *Design transfer* establishes and maintains procedures to transfer into production specifications.

– *Design change* documents how design changes are identified and validated. Design change is a procedure to be set up before implementation of any changes and must anticipate future changes in the product. Changes during the premarket review or during an Investigational Device Exception review must be reported to the FDA. All design changes will be recorded in the *Design History File*.

The *Design History File* sums up records describing the design history and the finished design. The document should take advantage of paper or electronics lab books (e.g. LabGuru).

EXAMPLE OF INFUSION PUMP.–

Infusion pump stops operating in the vicinity of high-voltage medical devices.

Questions to consider are as follows:

– What are the user needs?

– What is the environment for the infusion pump?

– What other kinds of equipment are nearby?

– What design input is needed to avoid this problem?

2.6. Risk management procedures (ISO 14711)

Risk management procedures for medical devices are mandatory for the European Union market. Standard recommendations are pooled in ISO 149711:2019 Medical Devices – "Application of Risk Management to Medical Devices". The risk management could concern, in particular, the design process, device production or conditions of use. Considering the complexity of medical device design, focused risk management practices help ensure usability, safety, and regulatory compliance.

Risk management gathers many concepts that must be clarified. First, the *risk management* itself is a systematic application of management policies, procedures and practices to analyze, evaluate, control and monitor *risk*; that is, the combination of probabilities of occurrence of harm and severity of the harm. The *harm* should be seen as an injury to people or damage to material or the environment. The *severity* of it is a measure (or an estimate) of the possible consequences.

Risk assessment consists of identifying hazards and estimating the risk from any available sources of information (*risk analysis*). A probability of occurrence of harm and a severity has to be assigned to the hazard (*risk estimation*); finally, the risk must be compared to a given criterion to determine its acceptability (*risk evaluation*). The initial risk can be mitigated by making decisions and implementing countermeasures (*risk control*), but of course, a complete safe situation is impossible, and a *residual risk* is always present.

Risk analysis should detect every risk source. Standard methods, such as hazard and operability (HAZOP) or failure mode effects analysis (FMEA) can be used. Anyway, risk analysis should consider major components and operational requirements such as raw materials (including wastes), hardware, monitoring and control systems, human–device interfaces and services. There are certain hazards that must be evaluated:

– raw materials and waste: flammability, toxicity, chemical reactivity, biocompatibility, etc.;

– environmental factors: temperature, moisture, vibrations, radiations, etc.;

– mechanical or electronic hazards;

– human factors: hazards due to lack of training, transmission of information, etc.

The risk estimation and evaluation are a complex task, as they combine well-defined considerations and others that are experience-based. Discussions with end users (practitioners and patients) and bibliographical research (evaluation of similar products[5], standard and guidance documents) are helpful. When the probability and severity are stated for a given harm, the risk is estimated using a risk acceptability matrix (Figure 2.3). As it is a combination, the risk could be moderate, even if the severity of the harm is critical if the probability for this harm is negligible (improbable). For example, during a walk test, the patient can fall, hit their head on a piece of furniture, be injured and eventually suffer disability or even die. The probability of falling during the test in itself is low and if it is combined with a clinical procedure rejecting the presence of a piece of furniture near

5 The Maude database is an unavoidable source: https://www.accessdata.fda.gov/scripts/cdrh/cfdocs/cfmaude/search.cfm.

the pathway, the combined probability is close to zero, and so is the risk.

Risk control should be performed for every identified harm. An objective is to demonstrate that the risk level has been intentionally lowered. Reduction in the risk level can basically follow three paths: improving the design (safety by design), protective measures in the device itself or in the manufacturing process, and information and training for safety.

Actually, even if each individual risk is identified and minimized through the risk assessment procedure described above, a decision has to be made considering all the residual risks on the overall risk of the device. The acceptable risk level depends on many parameters, such as the device, technologies or even the company's risk acceptability policy.

Risk acceptability matrix

Probability \ Severity	Negligible	Minor	Serious	Major	Critical
Frequent	Moderate	Moderate	High	High	High
Probable	Low	Moderate	Moderate	High	High
Occasional	Low	Low	Moderate	Moderate	High
Remote	Low	Low	Low	Moderate	Moderate
Improbable	Low	Low	Low	Low	Moderate

Figure 2.3. *Risk acceptability matrix. For a color version of this figure, see www.iste.co.uk/molimard/biomedicaldevices.zip*

The risk management is reported in two documents: the risk management plan and a living risk management file. During the product lifecycle, the risk management process is fed by users' feedback, quality department reports, fault tree analysis after device failure, corrective and preventive action (CAPA), or audits.

Other documents such as design outputs, design verification and design validation can be used in the risk management at any stage of the process.

2.7. Conclusion

Designing a medical device is much more than designing a device. It includes most of the usual designing steps, but must add extra features for compliance to regulatory offices. This specific difficulty could make the project fail in the pre-market phase (i.e. medical device start-up "death valley"). A precise development strategy must be developed in order to define the targeted market (mostly a country) and, therefore, the regulatory framework.

This chapter presented the two main aspects of the European and North American markets, but other considerations must be taken into account, the most important being the conditions of entry into the social protection system to obtain the coverage of the medical device for patients.

PERSONAL PRACTICE.– A respiratory assist device consists of an air pump coupled to a mask through a valve; it is widely used in intensive care units. Clarify the environment, the input and output variables of the system, then establish a risk assessment for this device. Lastly, imagine solutions to reduce the risks and compare to the technical solutions already in use.

3

Medical Sensors

3.1. Selection of medical sensors

3.1.1. *Introduction*

Medical sensors are used in many surgical medical devices: endoscopic surgery tools, cardiac systems and insulin pumps. More recently, they have appeared to be key to new medical devices that seek to monitor health indicators for the patient or even for healthy people all of the time. But, behind smart devices or smartphone applications, the basis is a sensor, and so understanding how sensors work and how reliable they are is inevitable.

Studying all existing medical sensors would make up a whole book, as is the case in Brown et al. (1999). Here, we will focus only on only a few of them, leaving aside some very important applications that could have been described here: radioscopy and non-irradiating methods for imaging and image processing.

3.1.2. *Electric signalization*

Electric signalization is an important topic for body monitoring. It consists of electrocardiography (ECG), electromyography (EMG) and electroencephalography (EEG), which record signals from the heart, muscles or brain for the purpose of diagnosis. Electricity/body interaction can be used for treatment; for example, transcranial stimulation is proven to be efficient for depression and other possible diseases within the same scope (Parkinson's, Alzheimer's, insomnia, etc.). Electric signal recording and transmitting is the central technical part of future treatment for spinal cord injury patients, as developed at EPFL (Wagner et al. 2018), as well as in arm or leg prosthesis.

Physiological signals

Physiological electric signals propagate along neurons or muscular cells.

A neuron, at rest, is polarized, meaning that the charge is negative inside and positive outside. When a signal propagates across the axon (the neuron trunk), sodium pumps open and provoke an inversion of the polarity. This phase is followed by potassium pumps opening, we reverse the polarity, and the axon locally goes back to its initial state. Thus, the neuron signal consists of a rectangular function.

We must highlight the difference between myelinated and nonmyelinated neurons. Myelin is an insulator blanket with holes (nodes of Ranvier) that causes a speeding up of the electric propagation. A functional classification of neurons based on myelin is not easy, but myelinated neurons are mostly present in the peripheral and central nervous system and nonmyelinated neurons are found in the automatic nervous system.

As mentioned above, a signal propagates along the axon by a depolarization/repolarization phenomenon. This means that the intensity of the signal is determined by the neuron shape and the Na/K electro-chemical potential. The transmission of information with different levels is obtained by speeding up or slowing down a nervous impulse train.

Information is encoded by frequency modulation. In addition, in many cases, for example, vision, it is necessary to collect and transmit very low levels of information (luminance of 10^{-6} cd·m^{-2}, that is, a candle placed at a distance of 48 km!) and high levels of information (luminance of 10^{5} cd·m^{-2}). In such a situation, the signal is encoded in a logarithmic scale that smooths out this large variation. Finally, the impulse train has an amplitude from 50 to 100 mV, each impulse time is 1 ms and the impulse frequency can be as high as 5 kHz.

This change in the local polarity is not what is measured by an electrode. Usually, they are placed on the skin, outside of the body, but even in the case of micro-needles, some tissue separates the electric source and the electrode. Therefore, it is important to contemplate the tissues surrounding the electric transmitter, whether it is a neuron or a muscular cell. Evidently, the electrode catches potential variation from the targeted nerve or muscle, but also from other tissues or other events that may occur in the body (tribo-electricity of clothes, for example), in the sensor (potential between the electrode and the medium) or even outside (antenna effects from wires, ground loop).

It is possible to use a simple model to describe the electrical field around a neuron or muscular cell. If an element dx of a cylindrical cell is subjected to an intensity $I_m dx$, and if the medium around is homogeneous and infinite with resistivity ρ, the electric potential ϕ at a distance r is given by:

$$\phi(r) = \frac{\rho I_m dx}{4\pi r} \qquad [3.1]$$

The expression of the intensity I_m can be expressed in the nerve using intensity conservation:

$$I_m = \frac{2a}{\rho}\frac{d^2V}{dx^2} \qquad [3.2]$$

with a as the cylinder radius and V as the trans-membrane potential. Equations [3.1] and [3.2] show that ϕ is sensitive to the spatial variation of the potential V and not to the potential itself, so an equipotential situation would give no signal.

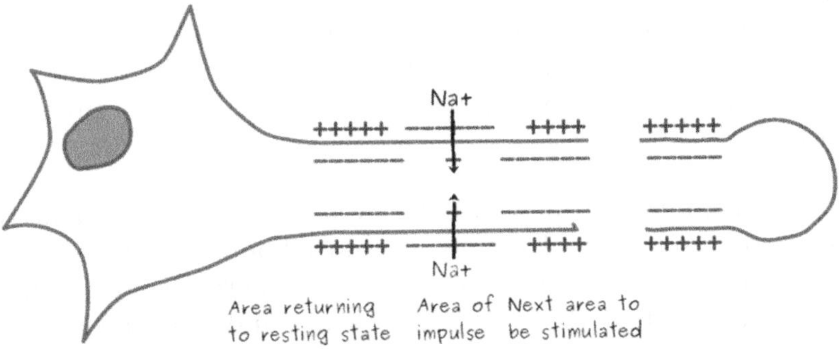

Figure 3.1. *Propagation of impulse along a neuron. For a color version of this figure, see www.iste.co.uk/molimard/biomedicaldevices.zip*

Electrodes

An electrode is basically an electrical conductor that can collect charges on a substrate, usually the skin, and transmit it to an electrical circuit that converts it to usable information, usually a tension. The conductor is a metallic part, and the interaction between the metal and the substrate creates a dipole with a potential that is usually higher than the potential rising from the body. The easiest way to remove most of this potential is to connect a pair of electrodes at two different points and stop their potential. The difference due to body effects will be recorded and the difference in the potential will be removed, but for many reasons, the potential at the two points should be slightly different and vary with time. This fluctuation is a source of noise. The silver/silver chloride type is considered to be the most stable arrangement.

If two electrodes are placed on the body with a potential between them, and an amplifier to record it, then a current should flow from one to the other, which results in a decrease in the potential to be measured. Therefore, the amplifier must have a high impedance (e.g. 1 MΩ for EEG). A typical arrangement for the amplification unit is shown in Figure 3.2 (right).

Finally, a direct contact between the metal surface and the substrate would be sensitive to movement that would result in changes in the contact resistance. Therefore, the best solution is to use a small cavity that is filled with electrolyte (Figure 3.2, left).

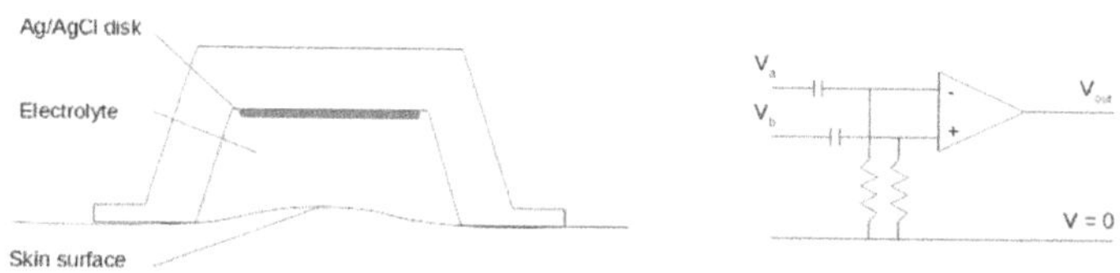

Figure 3.2. *Electrode (left) and its amplifier (right). For a color version of this figure, see www.iste.co.uk/molimard/biomedicaldevices.zip*

Applications

The application of electric signalization is a medical specialty, and explaining the details here would be unnecessary but, considering how easy it is to get a signal and the dynamics of start-ups aiming at mining electric signalization, highlighting the state-of-the-art precautions seems more than necessary.

ECG (or EKG) is the oldest detection method. On the one hand, the heart is internal and the only way to access the electric flux is to place electrodes around the trunk. On the other hand, the heart contraction pattern is complex, with the systolic and diastolic contraction sequence and a global twist of the heart inside the chest cavity.

Many electrode placements are used to investigate what happens in the heart, but these electrodes are external[1] and only obtain indirect information. Positions are normalized: left arm, right arm and left leg are used to study heart contraction in the frontal plane, but other implantations are used for the transverse and the sagittal plane.

Basic precautions must be taken for patient care. Electric leakages are made more dangerous by a transcatheter probe placed in the cardiac cavity, for example, for pressure monitoring or an external pacemaker. Then, it is even more important to correctly ensure the insulation of every system around the patient's bed.

In a very different area, electrodes are in contact with the skin. A bad choice of electrode can result in skin irritation because of material corrosion during the measurement and more so for long-term (ambulatory) monitoring. Silver-based electrodes and hypo-allergenic jelly can be used.

Recordings may be affected by interference coming from muscular contraction near the electrodes. These effects are even more important for stressed patients that may imagine an exam will be painful or simply be anxious about the results. A convenient signal filtering can remove most of the noise by selecting relevant frequencies or rejecting others (see section 4.2.2).

An electroencephalogram records electrical activity from the brain. It is usually done on the skin of the skull, but some more invasive variants exist. Of course, being closer to the brain makes the signal interpretation easier, but the price for that is surgery. The main difficulty with EEG recordings is the amplitude of the signal (from 10 to 300 μV) compared to the noise (2 μV at best), therefore a good amplification is mandatory, even if it increases the signal as well as the

1 Except for the oesophagus electrode, which is used in the study of the sagittal plane.

noise. The best results are obtained using silver-based electrodes stuck with collodion and injected electrolyte jelly; a careful skin preparation must be done before (degreasing, then skin abrasion). Since this method is time consuming, most applications use saline pad electrode skullcaps. The classical 10–20 arrangement gathers 17 electrodes.

Because of the low amplitude of the signal, many artifacts can pollute the information. They both originate in the technical aspects and the patient. As an example, technical problems can arise if the environment is electromagnetically polluted, or if the patient wears a pacemaker, or even due to the presence of dental fillings. During the test, the patient must be as quiet as possible: any muscular activity (eye movements, abnormal ventilation, etc.) could generate artifacts.

Procedures for EEG recording are therefore restrictive: they must take place in an acoustically and electrically quiet room, far away from electromagnetic noise sources (e.g. surgery theater); only one person can be in the room with the patient. The patient has to relax for 5–10 min with their eyes closed, then open their eyes and keep relaxing. Following this, depending on the study, the patient may be asked to hyperventilate or be subjected to a flashing light (15 Hz). Conventionally, EEG signals are classified according to their frequencies: δ waves $\leq$ 3 Hz, θ waves $\in$ [3 Hz, 7 Hz], α waves $\in$ [7 Hz, 14 Hz], β waves > 14 Hz.

Finally, EMG is used to follow muscular and neural behavior. A muscular unit has its own electric signature, but cannot be recorded alone. The muscle recruits progressively muscular fibers – made up of muscular units – making the signal generated by a muscle complex. Again, electrodes are usually placed on the skin after careful preparation (degreasing and skin abrasion). The recording corresponds to the studied muscle, but with a contribution from other components (neurons or muscles). In addition, skin usually does not move as the muscles do when a large movement is performed, making interpretation more difficult. Needles or fine wire electrodes can be used to catch information closer to the muscle, but this method is invasive.

A typical arrangement consists of two electrodes that record activity between one another. They might be placed at the two ends of a muscle, but the signal will integrate more than this single muscle information. Bipolar needle electrodes can be used alone and give more local information, but the signal will be of lower amplitude and higher frequency.

Again, analysis and interpretation of the signals is still a question for medical specialists and no routine signal processing is yet available. EMG equipment usually includes a neural stimulation unit that provokes the muscular contraction, making possible the measurement of the nerve conduction speed. It usually includes a loudspeaker that converts muscular signals into sound, with hearing being a very powerful way to analyze the signal signature.

	Amplitude	**Pulse time**	**Frequency band**
Neuron	50–100 mV	1 ms	? → 5 kHz
Brain	0.01– 0.3 mV		0.5 → 40 Hz
Muscle	2 mV	50 ms	10 Hz → 1 kHz
Heart	1 mV	Contraction cycle ~250 ms Refractory period ~250 ms	1 Hz → 100 Hz (diagnosis) 1 Hz → 40 Hz (monitoring)

Table 3.1. *Electric signal characteristics of the main body organs*

Finally, Table 3.1 summarizes the electric signals characteristics from neurons, the brain, muscle and the heart. The neuron case is taken apart, frequency bands overlap and a clear demultiplexing of frequency is not easy. In this context, the amplitude clearly shows how complex it is to extract a convenient brain signal.

3.1.3. *Thermal measurement*

Temperature in the human body is a marker of the metabolism and inflammatory process: the body's normal temperature should be 37 ± 0.8°C, but temperature could decrease down to 32°C in the arms. Therefore, the temperature should be taken inside the body, or as close as possible to it. Usually, it can be taken with precaution inside the mouth or the ears. Many sensors are sensitive to temperature. Here, we will focus on two electronic sensors and one optical sensor.

Thermistor

The resistivity of many materials changes with temperature, so probing the resistivity of a sensor is a way to estimate its temperature. The resistivity/temperature dependence is generally nonlinear. The integration of these sensors is done by using a Wheatstone bridge as presented in Figure 3.3. Considering the nominal resistance such as $R_{th} = R_2 = R_3 = R_4$, the output tension should be null. In case of a small resistance variation $\Delta R \ll R_{th}$, the output tension V_{out} is given by:

$$V_{out} = \frac{V_S \cdot \Delta R_{th}}{4 \cdot R} \qquad [3.3]$$

A fifth variable resistor can be added to the others in order to change the zero-state of the Wheatstone bridge and to linearize the overall sensor output to the temperature. A thermistor can finally give the temperature with a standard of 0.1°C.

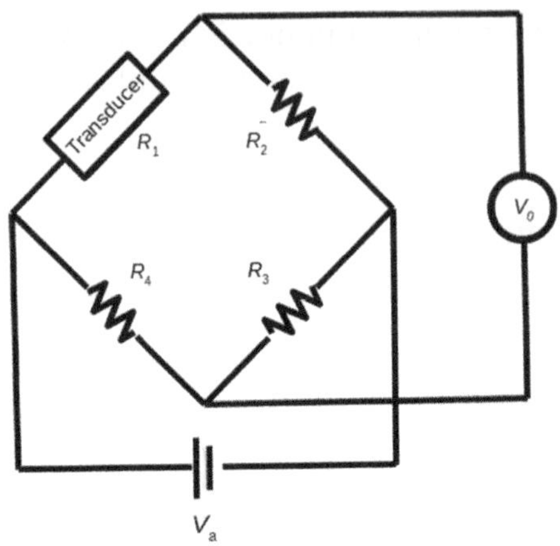

Figure 3.3. *Thermistor inserted into a Wheatstone bridge*

Thermocouple

When a bimetallic junction is subjected to a temperature change, a gradient of electric charges proportional to the temperature variation is created (Seebeck effect).

This tension can be amplified and measured. It is necessary to have a reference thermocouple giving a reference temperature. This second probe can be immersed in an ice/water melt or put on a Peltier cell. Thermocouples are classified depending on the couple of the metals, which corresponds to a different range of temperatures (Figure 3.4). For health applications, type J (iron/constantan) and type E (chromel/constantan) are good candidates, their typical range being from –40 to 750°C.

A thermocouple is a low-cost solution, with a reasonable measurement error, typically 0.1°C. The main error sources are the reference temperature that directly provokes a bias and the quality of the amplification that of course will also amplify noise.

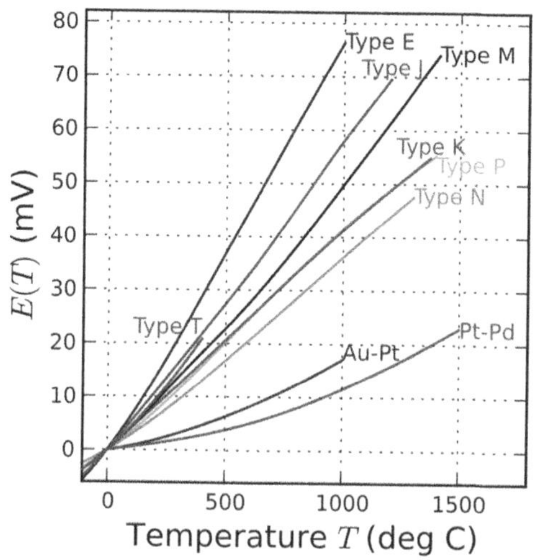

Figure 3.4. *Seebeck effect for various types of thermocouple (© user: Nanite/Wikimedia Commons/CC0 1.0). For a color version of this figure, see www.iste.co.uk/molimard/biomedicaldevices.zip*

Infrared measurement

Temperature measurement using infrared sensors was developed very rapidly. One of the major advantages of optical methods is that they are contactless, thus increasing prophylaxis and decreasing pain. Infrared thermometers determine the temperature of the object to be measured from the infrared radiation emitted by the body. The determination of the temperature is based on the radiation laws formulated by Planck. Let us consider a perfect black body, and its spectral radiance B_λ is given by:

$$B_\lambda(\lambda, T) = \frac{2hc^2}{\lambda^5} \frac{1}{e^{hc/(k_B \lambda T)} - 1} \quad [3.4]$$

where k_B is the Boltzmann constant, h is the Planck constant and c is the speed of light in the medium (the air).

The spectral radiance means a radiance for a given wavelength λ and absolute temperature T that follows $T|_K = T/_{°C} - 273.149$; the radiance being a quantity of energy emitted per unit of area and unit of solid angle. The spectral radiance unit is $W{\cdot}sr^{-1}{\cdot}m^{-3}$.

The study of Planck's law shows that the spectral radiance has an optimum that depends on the temperature. Figure 3.5 shows Planck's law at the temperature of the human body. The maximum radiance is reached for λ = 9.34 µm, that is, in the long-wavelength infrared. This corresponds to the sensitivity range of bolometers and micro-bolometers that are used in thermal cameras.

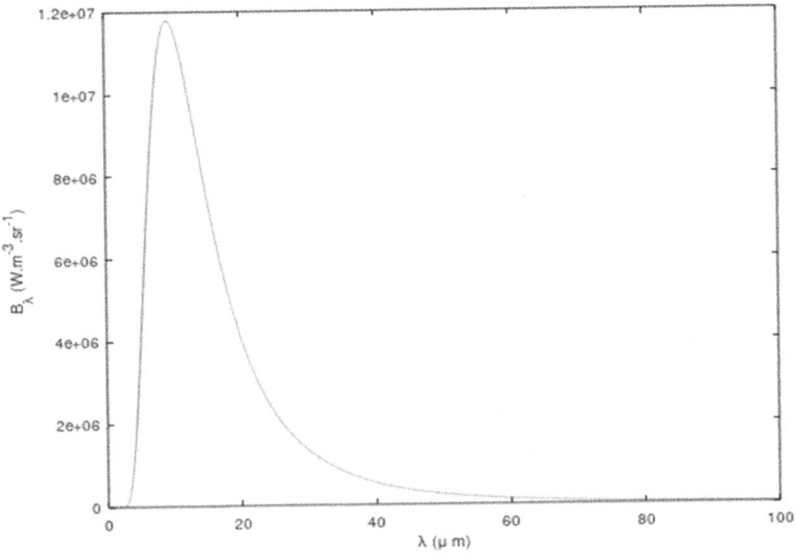

Figure 3.5. *Planck's law at human body temperature. For a color version of this figure, see www.iste.co.uk/molimard/biomedicaldevices.zip*

If equation [3.4] is integrated on the spectrum and the solid angle, the well-known Stefan–Boltzmann law is proposed. It states that the total energy emitted by a body is proportional to the temperature to the power of four.

Photometry describes and quantifies all of the processes, from energy emission of a surface to the collection on another surface: first, the radiation is emitted by an object in every direction in space. At a given distance, the radiation intercepts a surface defined by its orientation referring to the source. This gives an energy density and a total energy on the receiving surface. In the case of a sensor, this surface is covered by a sensitive element that transforms the radiation into an electrical signal that can be processed into a temperature later using a look-up table.

Then, the energy received by the detector is the radiation of a black body integrated over a *certain* surface both of the emitter and of the receptor, a *certain* solid angle, all of this depending on the geometrical arrangement, and on a *certain* frequency band that is related to the receptor properties and to the optical element transparency to these wavelengths.

Unfortunately, the black body is a model stating that the energy is completely emitted, but for real surfaces, part of the energy is stored, meaning that the transfer is incomplete. The ratio between the energy emitted and the total energy is the emissivity ε, $0 \leq \varepsilon \leq 1$. If the emissivity is constant over wavelengths, the surface is called a "gray body", but in some situations the emissivity changes with the wavelength. In addition, the Planck formula does not make any difference with the angle to the normal of the surface (Lambertian diffusion), but emissivity usually changes with the orientation.

Now, in a normal state, the skin's emissivity is 0.96 ± 0.03. This value changes however because of the biologically complex nature of the skin: physical activity or skin moisture changes the emissivity (Owda and Salmon 2019).

Emissivity changes near injuries, and thus may change the severity assessment (Keenan et al. 2017).

In addition to the radiation emitted by the surface of an object, an infrared detector also captures reflected radiation from the environment, or even infrared radiation that passes through the measured body. The arrangement around the camera or the sensor is therefore important.

3.1.4. *Biomechanical measurements*

Biomechanics covers many different items. Historically, the first biomechanical measurements were related to human movement, for rehabilitation or sports, but biomechanics also concerns strain and force measurement. One of the oldest works on this topic was that of Étienne-Jules Marey, who invented the chronophotograph in 1867. This first very important result was a temporal representation of the segment angular position (Figure 3.6).

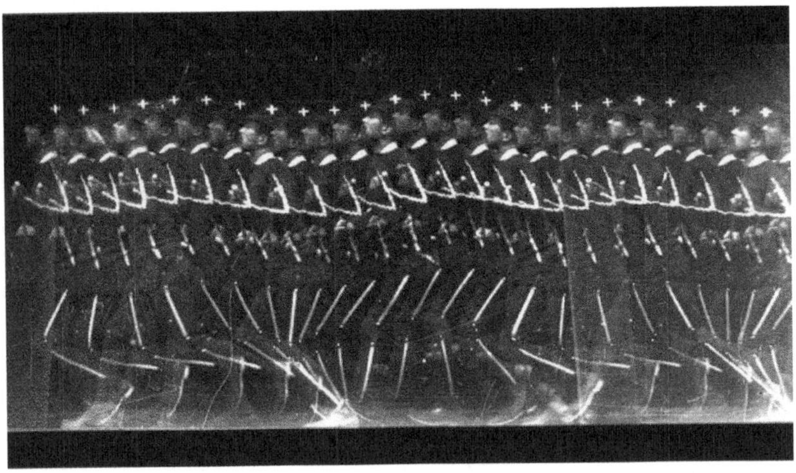

Figure 3.6. *Human walk by Étienne-Jules Marey (Coll. Cinémathèque Française) obtained at his physiological station in Paris (Marey 1883)*

Video recording of movements

Pioneering work from É.J. Marey opened the way to a huge quantity of applications and technical developments (including cinematography, with others, including E. Muybridge). Of course, using modern cameras was the first step toward video recording, replay and the automatic recording of points of interest. This recording can be based on a local thresholding and centroid detection. In this case, reflective markers or electroluminescent diodes are placed at the points of interest and result in white points in the image. Digital image correlation is another classical way of registration. A pattern I_1 in a reference image is sought in the current image by comparing to any pattern I_2 using a similarity criterion that can be written as:

$$P(r_0, s_0, T) = \frac{\sum_{r_0-\Delta r}^{r_0+\Delta r} \sum_{s_0-\Delta s}^{s_0+\Delta s} [I_1(T\{M(r,s)\}) - I_2(M(r,s))]^2}{\sum_{r_0-\Delta r}^{r_0+\Delta r} \sum_{s_0-\Delta s}^{s_0+\Delta s} I_1(T\{M(r,s)\}) \cdot \sum_{r_0-\Delta r}^{r_0+\Delta r} \sum_{s_0-\Delta s}^{s_0+\Delta s} I_2(r,s)} \qquad [3.5]$$

where $M(r_0, s_0)$ is the reference point and T is the mechanical transformation that should account for translation, rotation and global strain tensor.

In this case, no specific white markers are required, but the zone where the measurement is expected must have enough information (contrast and frequency content). Many free pieces of software are based on one or the other principle[2].

However, the use of a single camera does have some limitations: any movement out of the plane of the optical sensor would result in an erroneous in-plane displacement

2 See, for example, Kinovea (https://www.kinovea.org/) or Tracker (https://www.physlets.org/tracker/).

due to the camera focal length. This limitation is overcome using a system with multiple cameras that can reconstruct the stereo-vision.

Multiple cameras are also necessary to catch information on any part of the body. This gives the modern gold standard in motion capture: a set of 8–12 infrared cameras tracking reflective markers[3]. Figure 3.7 shows a typical arrangement.

A huge amount of literature is available on this technique (see, for example, Chèze 2016) in biomechanics and more recently in animated movies. Application in health requires precautions in the use of motion capture. A careful calibration must be performed when any change occurs on the system. This calibration will identify each camera position (extrinsic parameters) and each camera lens distortion and focal length (intrinsic parameters). As in any measurement system, the range – here the field of view and therefore the density of markers – must be adapted to the study in order to maximize the signal-to-noise ratio. Then the system gives a displacement of markers that are stuck to the skin. Usually, what is sought is the skeleton movement, therefore a marker placement rule should lie on the minimum difference between skin movement and bone movement. In practice, recommendations on marker placement are given by system suppliers or universities.

Recently, some applications based on smartphones, Kinect or other low-cost systems have been published. As they are all based on optics as presented above, the precautions remain the same.

3 The most commonly used systems may be Vicon (https://www.vicon.com/), Motion Analysis (https://www.motionanalysis.com/) and Optitrack (https://www.optitrack.com).

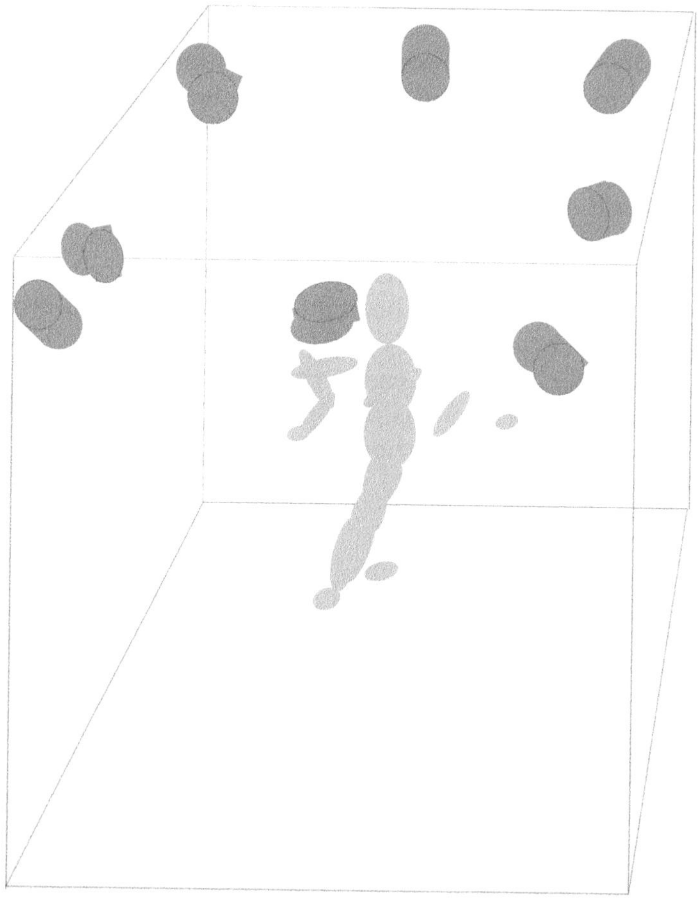

Figure 3.7. *Motion capture set-up: eight cameras (in blue). Subject (in orange) must be within calibrated volume. For a color version of this figure, see www.iste.co.uk/molimard/biomedicaldevices.zip*

Inertial measurement units

Recently, inertial measurement units (IMU) have appeared and have been used in health monitoring. IMUs gather a three-axis accelerometer with a three-axis gyroscope (6 degrees of freedom). A three-axis magnetometer is usually added to the system to give an IMU with 9 degrees of freedom. These sensors directly derive from the microelectronics industry, which gives low-cost high production systems, and are installed in smartphones or smartwatch. IMUs must be connected to a micro-controller that collects, processes and transmits data. Figure 3.8 shows two different approaches of the same sensor: on the left, a packaged sensor provided by an industrial supplier, here Awinda Xsens, that smooths out all low-level programing and communication tasks (the main drawback being a higher price and maybe limited access to the latest technology); on the right, a solution based on open electronics with a BNO055 IMU and an Adafruit Feather micro-controller. In this case, the user can better adapt the material to their needs, but must tackle more technical problems including calibration tasks.

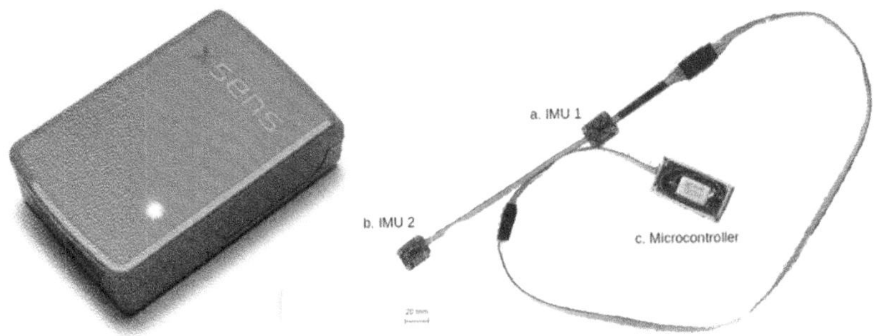

Figure 3.8. *Left: integrated IMU sensor (source: Awinda Xsens, Movella, the Netherlands). Right: Project specific development based on two BNO055 IMU and Adafruit Feather micro-controller. For a color version of this figure, see www.iste.co.uk/molimard/biomedicaldevices.zip*

Firstly, a three-axis accelerometer gives accelerations in a frame of reference corresponding to the sensor. The three-axis gyroscope measures rotation speed in the sensor frame of reference. Finally, the magnetometer gives as a result the projection of the magnetic vector along the sensor frame of reference. In the first implementation of IMUs, the question of the relative position of each sensor with respect to the others was important, but in the most recent implementations, the three sensors are integrated on the same chip and the frame of reference is unique.

Now, measurement outputs are in a local frame of reference that moves dramatically with respect to the world frame of reference. Unfortunately, raw data are often not convenient and prior to any other consideration; the data must be presented in the world frame of reference. This one is defined using first the accelerometer (at rest, the 1g acceleration corresponds to gravity) and the magnetometer. A magnetic field drift compensation may be added to get the absolute orientation. The classical AHRS algorithm from Madgwick et al. (2011) is presented in Figure 3.9. When movement begins, the orientation and the acceleration vector denoted as q at time t is known as a function of the orientation and the acceleration at time $t - \Delta t$, the angular velocity vector s_{ω} combined with the acceleration vector $s_{\hat{a}}$ in the local frame of reference integrated over Δt. This flowchart is indeed simplified, for it does not take into account the magnetic distortion compensation and the rotation drift.

Going from acceleration in the world frame of reference to the position is again a difficult task that still remains unusual because acceleration bias will lead to nonrepresentative displacements and usually comparisons between motion capture and IMUs are based on accelerations.

In any case, very interesting applications using a complete set of sensors have been developed under the form of active suits. Calibration is necessary to get the patient structure and positions are extracted from a body model and rotation vectors. This tool has given applications in ergonomics.

Indeed, many applications use low-level data (acceleration and rotation speed) as a signature to discriminate a movement (sit-to-stand, fall, etc.) or a pathology (Parkinson, aging, etc.).

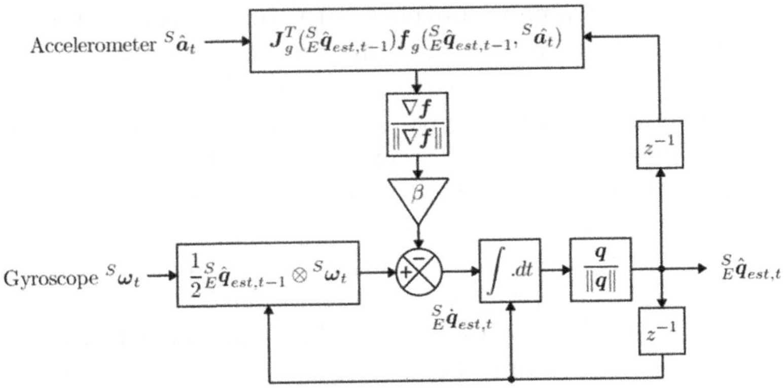

Figure 3.9. *Simplified AHRS algorithm flowchart from Madwick et al. (2011)*

Strain and force measurement

The force measurement is common in classical biomechanics and is useful for gait analysis (force plates), frailty assessment (grip) or sports biomechanics. Force in itself cannot be measured: a strain (sometimes a displacement) is measured on a test body that has known stiffness.

Classical design can be presented in Figure 3.10 (left). The central arm deforms in flexion and this flexion is measured using strain gauges. The load applied to these sensing elements changes its resistance, which are recorded through a Wheatstone bridge (see Figure 3.10, right). The S-shape is only one example of test body and it could also be a beam, a membrane, a torus, etc. Depending on the design, the load cell response can be more or less linear and the deflection can be more or less pronounced. All of the load cells are sensitive to overloading, but some protective elements can be included into the design. The total weight is important in dynamic applications and limits the frequency range. To reach the highest frequencies, a crystal-based load cell must be used. In this case, the measurement consists of collecting the electrostatic charges that are generated by the crystal on the loaded faces. The sensor acts as a capacitor, but this technology lacks stability along time and must be limited to dynamic applications.

Since the force is a vector, it is worth mentioning that the load cell only captures a scalar, that is, the projection of the force vector along the load-cell sensitivity vector. In the case of resistivity-based sensors, the error remains that of the projection, but it is more complicated in the case of capacity-based sensors, where the electric charges are not collected properly.

A load cell is simple and robust and can be used in many applications but apparent strain may vary according to environmental conditions (temperature). A specific arrangement of the strain gauges can limit this drawback. In any case, the load cell has to be calibrated before use and, as with any sensing element, a calibration with a standard is required at least once a year.

Accelerometers and pressure sensors are directly derived from load cells. Accelerometers measure the deformation of the test body equipped with an inertial element.

Pressure sensors are usually small hemispheric shells that bend when pressure is applied. Another technology for pressure measurement consists of measuring the resistivity variation of a foam. This is the basic principle of resistivity-based pressure mapping systems. The foam can be replaced by a semiconductor arrangement and a capacity is measured instead of a resistance. These two arrangements have their particularities: capacity-based mapping systems are very sensitive to bending when resistivity-based systems are not; resistivity-based systems have some viscoelastic effects due to the use of a foam (Bonnaire et al. 2014).

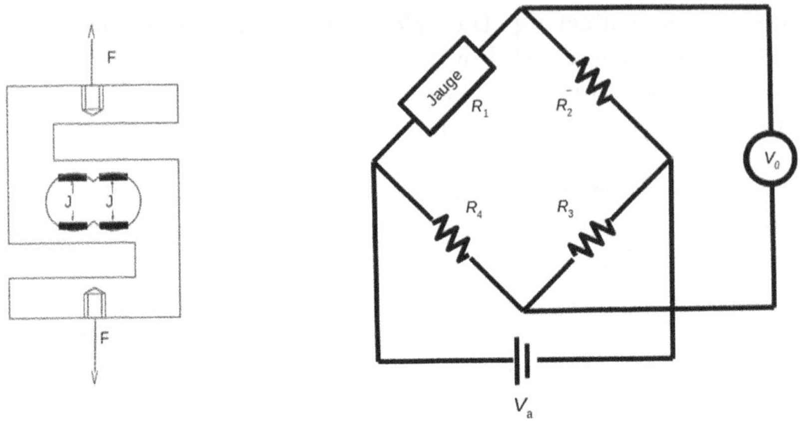

Figure 3.10. *Left: S-shape load cell (adapted from Molimard (2016))*

3.1.5. *Exercises*

Falling of elderly population

Propose three ways to detect the falling of elderly people. Each proposition should describe the physical principle, the sensor conditioning and a discussion on advantages and drawbacks.

Force/strain measurement: understanding the Wheatstone bridge

From Figure 3.10, write the potential V_0 as a function of V_a and R_i, $i = 1...4$. Simplify the system with (1) all resistors equal to R, one of them undergoing a small variation δR, (2) $\delta R << R$.

Hint: You should consider the Wheatstone bridge as a two-arm system with the same potential V_a and calculate the potential at each resistor end.

4

Measurement Quality

4.1. Measurement quality[1]

4.1.1. *Introduction*

Despite all the efforts that can be made to increase measurement quality – including the associated signal processing – medical sensors inevitably give some measurement errors, and a measurement is always an imperfect representation of reality. It is necessary to be able to estimate the errors to produce an experimental result and no result should be given without its range and the level of probability accorded to it.

Of course, measurement errors (and more the random part of it) enter into the discussion on statistical testing. It is usually legitimate to argue on the inter-subject variability, but if the medical device uses a sensor as a key part, then this sensor has to be carefully checked in order to validate its use (and to check underlying assumptions) and to increase the medical device quality. This happens frequently in the context of small electronic devices within the IoT family, where most of the efforts are put into the software and numerical methods from artificial intelligence.

1 This section is partly derived from Molimard (2016). The reader might refer to this book for a more in-depth understanding.

4.1.2. *Calibration*

Calibration aims to give a correspondence table or a function between the value given as an output of the sensor (in general, a potential difference) and the measurand (e.g. a load). Calibration becomes necessary if the acquisition model is too complex and/or if the variables that need to be known in the model are poorly known. For example, a load cell can very often be modeled using beam theory, but there are many reasons to move away from this simple analytical model. These can relate to the model's limits (e.g. assumptions on the stress field and quality of clamping) or to the test conditions (e.g. geometrical misorientation and temperature).

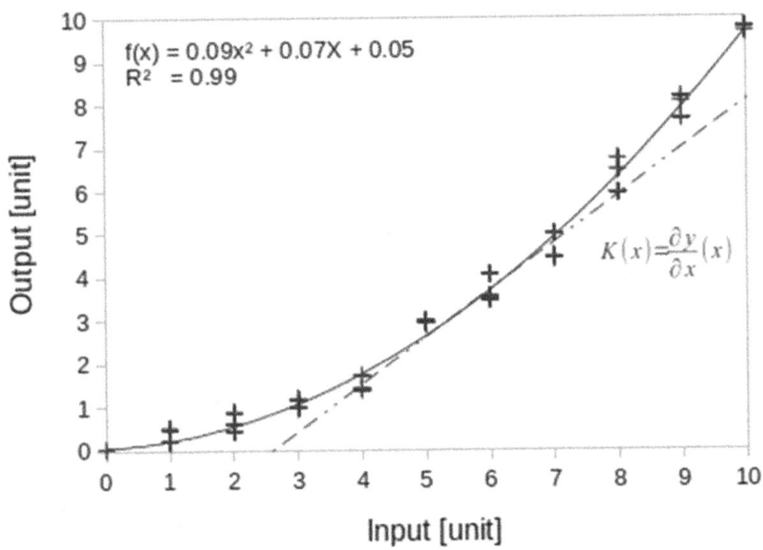

Figure 4.1. *Typical calibration curve. For a color version of this figure, see www.iste.co.uk/molimard/biomedicaldevices.zip*

This calibration can be made at the sensor level or for the entire measuring chain. Before calibrating, it is important to identify the quantities that could influence the output and to take them into account in the context of a multi-variable calibration, or by adding corrective terms. The environment parameters, such as the temperature or the degree of hydrometry, often have an influence, especially if the sensing part is made up of polymers. Similarly, time and frequency are critical parameters. Above the cut-off frequency, the sensor will not be capable of returning information and the response will be erroneous, even for lower frequencies close to the cut-off frequency. Lastly, a calibration will be valid within a certain experimental domain, that of the measurand or that of influence factors; therefore, calibration has to be carried out in the conditions in which the sensor is used.

Figure 4.1 shows a typical calibration curve, with several important elements. First of all, the *measurement points* appear "reasonably *dispersed*". To quantify this dispersion, it is necessary to give a reference curve (*calibration curve*), obtained by smoothing the previous values. This operation is carried out correctly if the smoothing function is well chosen. Is it necessary to use a straight line? What theoretical or practical consideration can we rely on? A defect in form in the smoothing function would lead to a systematic error on the values measured later on. The average difference between the points and the curve therefore becomes a dispersion of the measurement. Finally, the slope $K(x)$ at any point on the calibration curve corresponds to the measurement system's *sensitivity*.

4.1.3. *Vocabulary*

The International Bureau of Weights and Measures defines various concepts around measurement, as precision in terms is particularly important (BIPM 2012). For all of the scientific community, it is important to stick to this vocabulary to have a good interdisciplinary understanding.

– *Measurement error* is the difference between the measured value of a quantity and a reference value.

– *Measurement accuracy* is the closeness of the agreement between the average of an infinite number of repeated values measured and a reference value. Accuracy in itself cannot be expressed numerically. It varies in inverse direction to the systematic error, a component of the measuring error which, in repeated measurements, remains constant or varies predictably. Systematic error is estimated by a *bias*.

– *Random error* is a component of the measuring error which, in repeated measurements, varies unpredictably. Measurement precision takes account of the random error, depending on the method chosen, the conditions of *repeatability*, conditions of intermediary precision or conditions of *reproducibility*. Precision is usually expressed by a standard deviation, a variance or a variation coefficient.

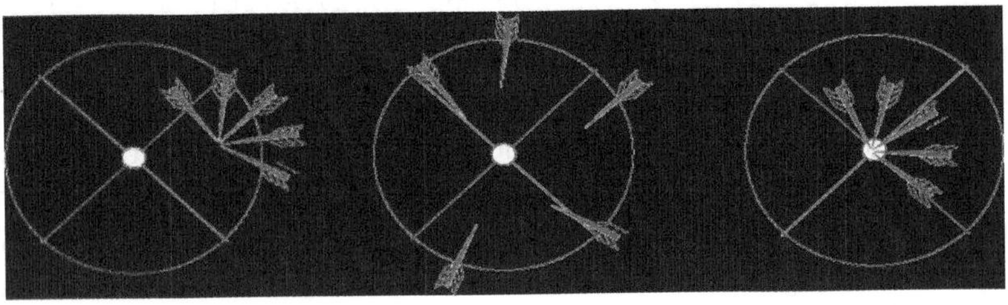

Figure 4.2. *Illustration of trueness and precision. For a color version of this figure, see www.iste.co.uk/molimard/biomedicaldevices.zip*

Trueness and precision can be illustrated using the darts in Figure 4.2. In the first instance, the launcher is extremely reproducible, but there is an error in trueness (darts are not in the center of the target). In the second instance, the precision is weaker, although the darts are generally well centered. These two cases give a measurement accuracy of the same order of magnitude, but the reality is very different. Evidently the third situation is the best; however, this case is not always preferred, because the cost of instruments usually increases with precision.

These definitions should not be confused with the definition that quantifies, using the errors defined above, the reasonable range of variability in a specific measurement.

4.1.4. *Metrological testing*

Finally, the definitions of the different kinds of errors given above classify them in a mathematical meaning, between random errors and systematic errors. In practice, various metrological tests exist, either sequential or random, in order to characterize these errors. All these tests help to establish the *instrument's total error*, estimated as the quadratic mean of all the errors that could be identified.

Sequential tests

Sequential tests are tests used to reveal historical phenomena in the measurement; this effect can be directly related to time or whatever physical quantity has changed over time (load, pressure, etc.).

– *Drift* is quantified by maintaining a constant situation over time and observing the long-term variation of the indicator.

– *Hysteresis* is the gap that could be observed between the ascending and descending curves. This indicates an energy dissipation in the measurement system, for example, dry friction or viscoelasticity. A hysteresis test consists of the successive acquisition of a given output by incrementally changing the input from the smallest value to the uppermost and then back to the smallest. Figure 4.3 shows an example in the case of foam-based pressure sensors. Since this foam has a relaxation time, the return path is not the same as the initial one. Hysteresis error is defined as the maximal gap Δy between the values found in each direction over the maximal value y_{max}:

$$e_{h_{max}}(\%) = \frac{\Delta y}{y_{max}} \times 100 \quad [4.1]$$

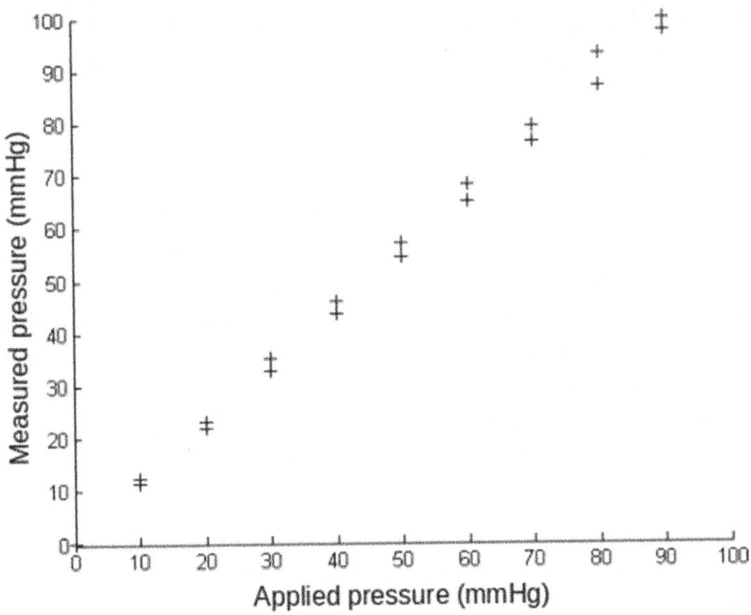

Figure 4.3. *Hysteresis testing of a pressure sensor*

Random tests

Random tests erase the historic effects and can detect linearity defects, sensitivity or the instrument's precision in intermediate precision conditions.

Assuming an affine relationship linking the measured signal and the measurand, *linearity* is usually defined by:

$$e_{linearity} = \frac{max(y-\widehat{y_{lin}})}{y_{max}} \times 100 \quad [4.2]$$

where $\widehat{y_{lin}}$ is the linearized value of the measurand[2]. This definition shows that linearity is related to the device's

2 Following the BIPM (2012), the measurand is the quantity intended to be measured.

range. Linear regression and the associated uncertainty will be developed in section 8.4.1.

Precision can be defined by different conditions, corresponding to different experimental concerns. In the first instance, *repeatability* is obtained with "the same measurement procedure, same operators, same measuring system, same operating conditions and same location, and replicate measurements on the same or similar objects over a short period of time" (BIPM 2012). However, these conditions are too strict to reproduce operating conditions, for example, the operator effect, the laboratory experience or habits or long time periods. *Reproducibility* covers various measuring conditions "includ[ing] different locations, operators, measuring systems, and replicate measurements on the same or similar objects".

Repeatability or reproducibility characterize statistical variables and are defined using a standard deviation σ as:

$$e_{precision} = \frac{2.\sigma}{y_{max}} \times 100 \qquad [4.3]$$

The last commonly used term, the resolution is the smallest change in a quantity being measured that causes a perceptible change in the corresponding indication. Resolution is thus related to precision, but usually resolution refers to the instrument whereas precision refers to the measurement, and then with many more factors that should be taken into account.

DISCRIMINATION THRESHOLD.–

Besides these definitions based on a statistical approach, a measuring system has a deterministic detectable minimum that could be linked to a graduation for the oldest systems or a digital sampler for the most recent ones. This minimum is the discrimination threshold, which should not be mixed up with precision, which can be defined as the minimum value of the measurand associated with a meaningful change. The precision can be characterized by a repeatability test, whereas the discrimination threshold corresponds to a monotonic variation in the measured data. Usually, in a modern instrument design, the discrimination threshold is smaller than the resolution.

4.1.5. *Evaluating uncertainties*

Introduction

Previous tests are individual contributions that can help in characterizing an instrument, but the uncertainty associated with a measurement is more complex than that: all the sources of uncertainty should be taken into account. The budget includes estimations of uncertainties in the quantities involved in the measurements, links between these quantities (in the form of covariance) and the type of probability density functions used.

The current objective of analysis consists of "characterizing the dispersion of values that could, reasonably, be attributed to the measurand" as expressed by the *Guide to the expression of uncertainty in measurement* from the Bureau International des Poids et Mesures (BIPM 2008). The sources of uncertainties can be linked to:

– the measurand, either because it is not completely defined or because the practical test is itself incomplete. For example, this is the case for problems with friction;

– the choice of measurement sample. Typically, this is what occurs with all natural material and even more with a human being;

– the test conditions (temperature and hygrometry). There are numerous examples in skin studies;

– the measuring instrument and how it is used: the user can introduce bias or the system can be imperfectly calibrated, as stated before;

– the signal pre-processing algorithm: the calculation approximations and hypotheses create uncertainties. Basic examples should be re-sampling values or filtering, but more tricky situations can be found, for example, an infrared camera records a radiative flux that can be interpreted as a temperature using Planck's law and many assumptions.

Analysis can only be developed fruitfully when the objectives of the tests carried out are well defined, when the experiment procedure is written and validated, when the data are established for pertinent experimental values and when the experimenters have some experience with the system components.

This is usually done in two situations: when a new measuring device – including prototype – is put into service (type A evaluation) or at design stage (type B evaluation).

Evaluating type A

Type A evaluation is based on metrological tests on an instrument that can characterize biases and random errors. Usually, the systematic error can be compensated, for example, by using a calibration table. However, random error still persists. In the case of a measurement where the systematic error is null, the value measured should be described:

$$x = \bar{x} \pm u_x(P\%) \qquad [4.4]$$

where $\bar{x}$ is the average value, u_x is the confidence interval and P is the probability level.

Metrological tests on repeatability or reproducibility can give a variance on the data and its square root, the standard deviation. To obtain a range at a given confidence level (in general, 95%), a statistical distribution is required for the measurements. On the basis of central limit theorem, the distribution is supposed to be Gaussian but, because the standard deviation is experimentally known for a limited number of experiments, the right statistic here is the Student's distribution. Then, equation [4.4] is written as:

$$x = \bar{x} \pm E_{\nu,P} S_x (P\%) \quad [4.5]$$

where the coverage factor $E_{\nu,P}$ is function of the number of statistical degrees of freedom for the metrological tests ($\nu = N - 1$, with N the total number of tests) and the confidence level. S_x refers to the standard deviation of the set of measurement results. As this standard deviation is not the true one, it is denoted S_x and not σ.

The number of degrees of freedom comes from the finite statistics definition of the mean and the variance:

$$\bar{x} = \frac{1}{N} \sum_{i=1}^{N} x_i \quad [4.6]$$

$$S_x^2 = \frac{1}{N-1} \sum_{i=1}^{N} (x_i - \bar{x})^2 \quad [4.7]$$

The estimate of the variance S_x^2 uses the estimate of the mean $\bar{x}$; therefore, 1 degree of freedom is used in this operation and the number of remaining degrees of freedom is $N-1$.

Some values of the Student's coverage factor are presented in Table 4.1 and the probability density function is shown in Figure 4.4. The evolution of factor $t_{\nu,95\%}$ with the number of degrees of freedom is not linear and decreases as ν increases. Figure 4.4 shows that tails are bigger for the Student's distribution, meaning that the probability of having a value far from the mean is higher in the Student's distribution, which is the normal law. This explains why the coverage factor is higher for the Student's distribution.

ν	$t_{95\%}$	$n_{95\%}$	ν	$t_{95\%}$	$n_{95\%}$
1	12.706	1.96	7	2.365	1.96
2	4.303		8	2.306	
3	3.182		9	2.262	
4	2.770		10	2.228	
5	2.571		11	2.201	
6	2.447		12	2.179	

Table 4.1. *Student's t-test and normal distribution*

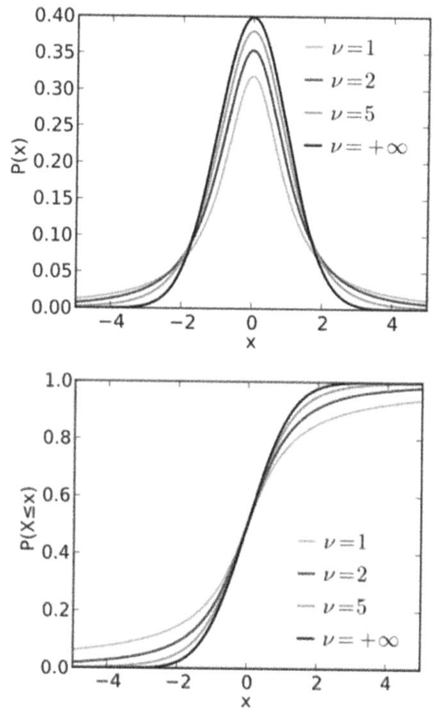

Figure 4.4. *Student's distribution for various degrees of freedom (source: Wikipedia). x is the reduced variable for (μ = 0, σ = 1). For a color version of this figure, see www.iste.co.uk/molimard/biomedicaldevices.zip*

Finally, equation [4.5] gives an estimate for each particular measurement, but what is the mean value if the measurement is repeated N times? Central limit theorem states that the experimental mean tends to the expected theoretical value, and the variance on the mean is given by:

$$S^2(\bar{x}) = \frac{S_x^2}{N} \qquad [4.8]$$

Type B evaluation

Type B evaluation should only be used when the first method is impossible, which is the case at design stage. This approach is based on scientific judgment using available data: the makers' specifications for equipment, the calibration certificate, the designer's experience or knowledge obtained from literature, etc.

If it is only possible to estimate a random variable's reasonable lower limit a^- and upper limit a^+, it is necessary to define a standard, that is, 1 standard deviation. A statistical distribution should be a uniform law and the value can take absolutely any of the values in this range, or a more complex distribution (triangular or trapezoidal law). The choice of the distribution depends on the type of sensors and display available; rules are given in BIPM (2008). The standard of a uniform distribution is given as:

$$u = \sqrt{(a^+ - a^-)/12} \qquad [4.9]$$

Standard is expressed for 1 standard deviation. In the case of normal law, it corresponds to a probability level of 68%, that is most often unsatisfactory and a level of 95% is often retained. Therefore, it is necessary to multiply the standard by a coverage factor to move from a confidence range of 68% to a confidence range of 95%, as already mentioned earlier.

Combining uncertainties

The different quantities influencing the measurement chain can be shown in a mathematical model, represented by a function f. By using a Taylor expansion for the function f and ignoring the higher order terms, equation [4.10] becomes linear, and it is possible to separate the deterministic and the random components:

$$\bar{y} = f(\bar{x}) \quad [4.10]$$

$$u_c^2 = \sum_{i=1}^{L}\left(\frac{\partial f}{\partial x_i} u_{x_i}\right)^2 \quad [4.11]$$

When the input data are correlated, it is necessary to take account of their interactions, that is, the extra-diagonal terms of the covariance matrix:

$$u_c^2 = \sum_{i=1}^{L} \left(\frac{\partial f}{\partial x_i}\right)^2 u^2(x_i) + 2\sum_{i=1}^{L-1}\sum_{j=i+1}^{L} \frac{\partial f}{\partial x_i}\frac{\partial f}{\partial x_j} u(x_i, x_j) \quad [4.12]$$

Monte Carlo method approach

Taylor series development is impossible if the signal-to-noise ratio is weak or if the parameters' dependence is very nonlinear. In this case, the propagation is modeled using numerical simulation.

The function describing the measurement chain represented by f should be expressed in an analytic or numerical form; f would then include the sources and appropriate statistical distribution and parameters must be decided. The Monte Carlo approach consists of launching a large number of random realizations of input parameters and writing the probability density function of the quantity to be measured. This analysis leads to the most probable value – the expected value – and the range of variation for a given level of probability – the expanded. The critical sources of those which most impact the measurements are also a very important result of this analysis.

4.2. Key notions in signal processing

Much signal processing can be applied on experimental data. A detailed view here would be completely beyond the scope of this book and the reader should refer to dedicated books. Only key elements will be given here.

4.2.1. *Signal sampling*

The signal, as sent by the sensor and its conditioner, is commonly a tension (AC or DC) continuous with time. Due to pre-processing and acquisition, this signal is transformed and sampled in two directions: first, it is time sampled, and data are recorded every Δt time period; second, it is intensity sampled, because digital acquisition boards are analog-to-digital (A-to-D) converters.

Figure 4.5 shows how the selection of sampling parameters can affect the signal. Firstly, the range of the sensor has to be carefully adapted to the measuring conditions in order to use as many intensity levels as possible and to get a detailed view on the measured factor. As the random error is proportional to the measuring range, an inadequate range would also result in a poor signal-to-noise ratio.

The sampling period is key in many applications. The sampling frequency or sampling rate is the inverse of the sampling period ($f_s = 1/\Delta t$). Again, the sampling period must be adapted to each device: if the sampling period is short, the quantity of data could be too high and result in storage and price issues. On the other hand, too long a time period will lose information. As an example, we may consider the IMUs presented in section 3.1.4 and the following. In posturography analysis, high frequency data (~ 200 hz) corresponding to muscular continuous dynamic correction are relevant and experiment duration is short (< 1 min), whereas daily activity monitoring needs only rough changes (sitting to standing changes, walking) over a long-time period: here, a 1 Hz frequency should be enough.

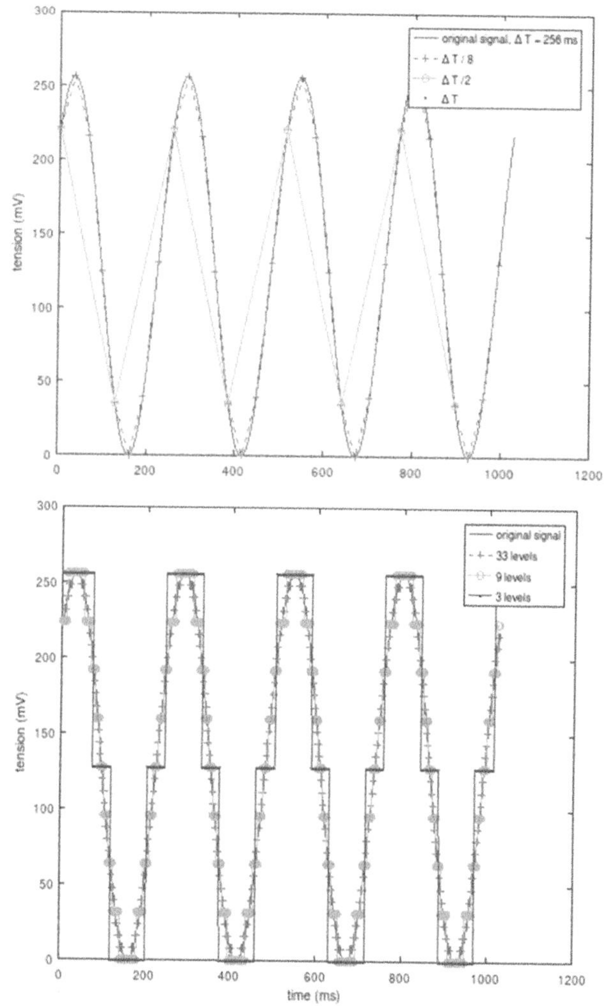

Figure 4.5. *Signal sampling with different time periods (left) or different encoding depths (right). For a color version of this figure, see www.iste.co.uk/molimard/biomedicaldevices.zip*

Selection of the highest frequency to be observed is a first step, but it is not *directly* the sampling frequency. In order to observe a given frequency from the experiment, the sampling frequency should be at least two times this frequency (Nyquist–Shannon theorem). Even in this condition, the signal can be modified due to *aliasing*, that is, the presence of a low-frequency effect of the sampled high-frequency components. This can be removed using a low-pass filter that reduces high-frequency components to noise level before sampling, but a low-pass filter provokes a change in the signal amplitude and phase near the cut-off frequency. A good filter should then preserve the frequencies lower than the cut-off frequency and decrease rapidly afterwards to reject higher ones. The quality of a filter is characterized by its order, and the capacity to reject high frequencies is the *filter stiffness*, given in decibel (dB) per octave. A lot of filters should be suitable, but the Papoulis–Legendre filter is known to be the most efficient.

4.2.2. Denoising a signal

Noise is frequently an issue when using large diffusion sensors, such as what happens sometimes in smartphone applications. Improving signal-to-noise ratio is possible, but the best solution is always to reduce noise before acquisition. The choice of the sensor is a first step; it has to be adapted to a given application, considering signal processing, and price issues. The sensor environment is a major source of noise; vibrations, electromagnetic perturbations and ground loops are the most common issues. In this context, temperature in many cases would give a drift (a bias) and not a random noise. Electromagnetic perturbations or ground loops can be prevented easily with circuit design, for example, by working on wiring (eight-shaped circuits, shielded cable); an appropriate A-to-D converter can avoid electromagnetic noise collection. In a normal situation, the noise level should be lower than one hundredth of the full range and the signal-to-noise ratio should not be lower than 3–10 in usual situations.

Noise should follow a classical probability distribution, usually normal (Gaussian) law or log-normal law, or should result in outliers. Even if the probability is close to zero, outliers might occur within a probabilistic distribution but very often, outliers can be directly related to identifiable events such as transmission errors or A-to-D errors. The detection of outliers is a delicate subject, because only erroneous points should be removed, but even less probable events containing information should be preserved.

Outlier detection is based on the probability of an event within a certain time period. Let us consider a series of measurements with sampling period Δt. The kth measurement can be compared with other measurements on a *certain* time period $t_k \pm \delta t_k$ where it can be considered that no major changes occur. Knowing the mean value and the standard deviation of surrounding points $\overline{M_k}, \sigma(M_k)$, the expected value for the measurement M_k should lie in the range $\overline{M_k} \pm t_{\nu,P}\sigma(M_k)$, with $t_{\nu,P}$ a coverage factor with probability level P. The probability of having the actual measurement M_k outside this range is $(1 - P)$, and it can be stated in this case that the point is doubtful. Then, the point can be discarded and might be replaced by a more probable value, the mean value or median value of surrounding points. Of course, this approach is based on a hypothesis of slow and regular variation, as that usually occurs in physics, but it would fail in case of bifurcations or instabilities.

Another more systematic way of removing outliers consists of replacing the actual value M_k by the median value calculated over a certain time period $t_k \pm \delta t_k$. Median value corresponds to the value with the same number of higher and lower values. Of course, in the case of an outlier, this value will be far from the median and will be removed; however, compared to the mean value, the median value is not perturbed by this outlier. This makes this way of filtering more robust to outliers. As a major drawback, the median filter tends to change values, even if it is not statistically justified, but the filter is usually implemented in numerical codes (Matlab/Octave, Excel/Calc, etc.) and runs quickly.

Outlier detection as well as median filter are nonlinear filters because they do not use a linear combination of the experimental points surrounding the value M_k. These nonlinear filters ought to be used before the linear filters that will be described below.

If the noise simply follows its probability distribution and if its level is too high for the interpretation that is sought, then it can be reduced with linear low-pass filters. In this case, each measurement M_k will be replaced by a weighted average of the surrounding points. The simplest way is to use the mean value over a horizon from $-h$ to $+h$. This is the *moving average* approach:

$$\overline{M_k} = \frac{1}{2h+1}\sum_{i=-h}^{i=h} M_{k+i} \quad [4.13]$$

Using weights w_i, a more general form will give:

$$\overline{M_k} = \frac{\sum_{i=-h}^{i=h} w_i M_{k+i}}{\sum_{i=-h}^{i=h} w_i} \quad [4.14]$$

or, in a vectorial form:

$$\overline{M_k} = (\cdots \quad w_i \quad \cdots)(\cdots \quad M_{k+i} \quad \cdots)' = W \cdot M_k' \quad [4.15]$$

If the noise is constant for the different measurement M_{k+i}, the noise reduction is given by:

$$var(\overline{M_k}) = var(M_k)WW' \quad [4.16]$$

As expression [4.14] shows, the weight vector $\boldsymbol{W}$ is a convolution window and inherits all the signal processing background related to it. It is worth noting here that:

– the convolution product is a simple product in Fourier domain;

– the convolution is not defined near the boundaries (if $h > k$ or $h + k >$ nb of measurements).

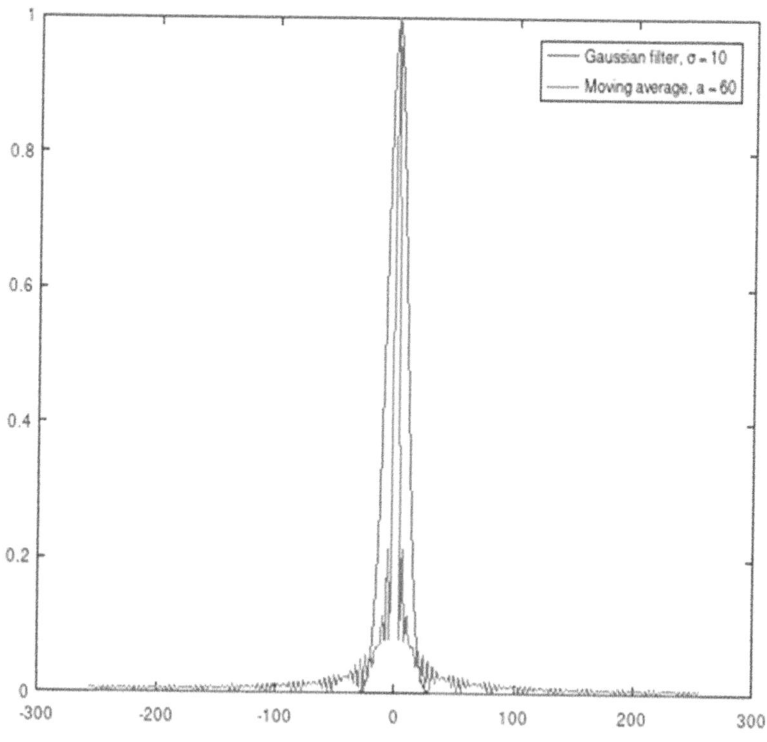

Figure 4.6. *Fourier transform of rectangular (moving average) and Gaussian filters. For a color version of this figure, see www.iste.co.uk/molimard/biomedicaldevices.zip*

This kind of filter is called a low-pass filter because it decreases the highest frequencies in the signal by temporally linking measurements; the quality of the filter is studied using its frequency signature. A very classical way to filter data consists of using Gaussian weights, because the Fourier transform of a Gaussian function is a Gaussian function; this means that no high frequencies will remain in the filtered signal, as Figure 4.6 shows. In this figure, the spectrum for a rectangular filter (with constant weight, as in the moving average case) and a Gaussian filter is presented. However, even if the frequency rejection is better for the Gaussian windows, Table 4.2 shows that the noise rejection is better for the moving average. The comparison between these two filters depends on their size. Here, the standard deviation of the two filters is the same, according to equation [4.9].

σ	Gaussian filter	Moving average
5	23.7×10^{-2}	13×10^{-2}
10	16.8×10^{-2}	9.2×10^{-2}
15	13.7×10^{-2}	7.5×10^{-2}
20	11.9×10^{-2}	6.5×10^{-2}
25	10.6×10^{-2}	6.2×10^{-2}

Table 4.2. *Noise reduction for Gaussian filter (σ) and moving average ($a = 6\ \sigma$)*

Finally, denoising can be performed in the frequency domain in the case of a good frequency separation between noise and signal. This is the case in particular if noise is of high frequency and the signal is of low frequency. Another frequent situation is a noise with a narrow frequency band, as it could be in case of interference (or 50/60 Hz power supply). Then, the signal can be projected on a sine/cosine basis:

$$\widetilde{M_k} = \sum_{n=0}^{N-1} M_n \cdot e^{-\frac{i2\pi}{N}kn} = \sum_{n=0}^{N-1} M_n \cdot [cos(-\frac{i2\pi}{N}kn) - i \cdot sin(-\frac{i2\pi}{N}kn)] \quad [4.17]$$

The amplitudes for frequencies that have to be removed can be set to zero. The corresponding phases might propagate artifacts; a random phase is usually sufficient to avoid this drawback.

4.2.3. *Time frequency representation*

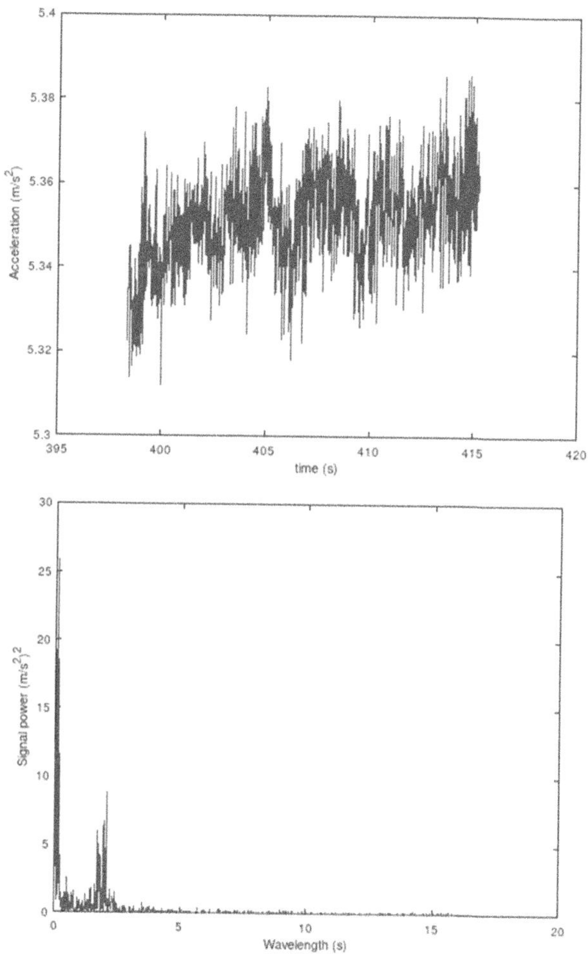

Figure 4.7. *Posturography output. Time result (left) and power spectrum (right). For a color version of this figure, see www.iste.co.uk/molimard/biomedicaldevices.zip*

As explained above, the Fourier transform is a classical way to visualize the frequencies present in a signal. As an example, the temporal result of a posturography test is shown in Figure 4.7. It is impossible to extract features and information from this signal, and two frequency domains arise from the Fourier transform of this signal: one at 0.5 Hz and other at 14 Hz. Even if the Fourier transform is a robust method that can give a lot of information, it has some limitations. Firstly, the Fourier transform implicitly states the periodicity of the signal and the signal continuity. This means that the signal at the beginning and at the end of the time scale should have the same amplitude. In its usual form, the fast Fourier transform, the time step between acquisitions must be constant. As a result, missing data draw difficulties and they have to be filled in some way. Finally, the result presented here is an average, over time, of all the data. We can imagine some changes in the frequency representation with time.

In gait analysis, for example, a change in the spectral signature is likely to indicate a change of posture (sitting to standing, walking to running, etc.). It would be useful to have another spectral representation for a limited period of time. As introduced earlier, the convolution product is the weighted sum of the signal moving from one point to the other. The convolution window could be rectangular or Gaussian for low-pass filtering. It can also be extended to many kinds of functions, and in particular to sine/cosine function, or in a more general way. Convoluting the signal on a set of short-term Fourier bases with different wavelengths gives, as a result, a Fourier transform at point t_0 that can be plotted as shown in Figure 4.8. The Fourier transform is represented along time, and it is possible to detect variations in the frequency distributions. Depending on the application, many functions with a real and orthogonal imaginary part, and with a scaling factor can be used as a wavelet. Most frequent forms are Gabor or Morlet wavelets.

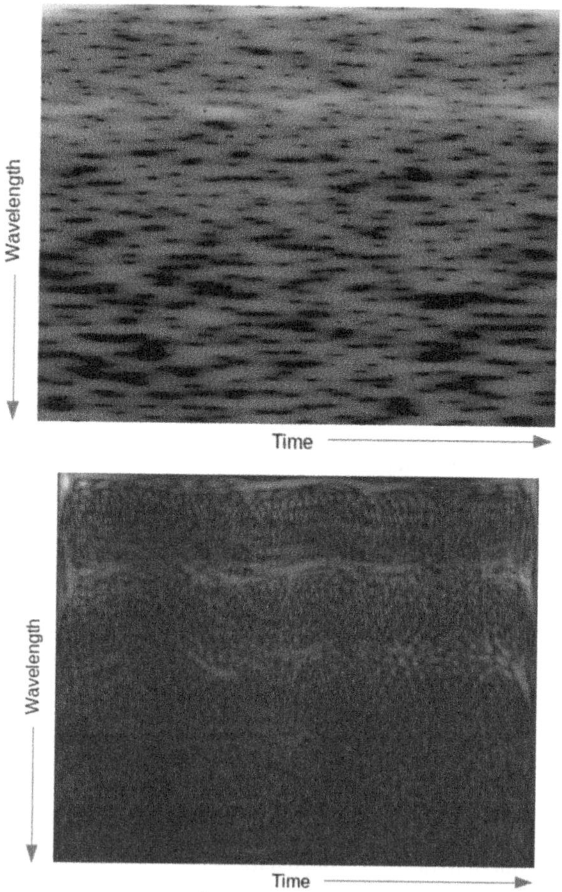

Figure 4.8. *Time-frequency representation (Posturography output). Left: Weigner-Ville transform. Right: Gabor wavelets. For a color version of this figure, see www.iste.co.uk/molimard/biomedicaldevices.zip*

4.2.4. *Extracting the information for high quantity of noisy data*

Biophysics representation is always complex and presents variability between subjects. For example, a leg shape is easily recognizable by a human being, but not by a computer. It would take a complete set of data for the computer to learn what a leg is and reproduce it. Principal component analysis

(PCA; also called proper orthogonal decomposition or Karhunen–Loève transform) should be helpful for that, but also for many more applications.

PCA is based on linear algebra; it is a way to represent a set of data on an orthogonal basis that best separates the different components. Let us consider a series of L experiments. Each experiment gathers N experimental data. As an illustration, if each experiment were an image, each piece of experimental data would be a pixel. Then, the set of experiments M (the knowledge we have on a problem) can be written as:

$$M = \left\{ \begin{matrix} X_{1,1} & \cdots & X_{1,N} \\ \vdots & \ddots & \vdots \\ X_{L,1} & \cdots & X_{L,N} \end{matrix} \right\} \qquad [4.18]$$

M can possibly be weighted on a quality criterion, and then centered and reduced. The normalization increases low-variation components; it could add noise, but it also reduces the mathematical instability of the covariance matrix.

$$\underbrace{\bar{M}}_{\text{center-reduced data}} = \frac{1}{W}\Big(\underbrace{M}_{\text{rough data}} - \underbrace{\frac{M^T \tilde{1}}{W}}_{\text{weighted gravity center}} \Big) \qquad [4.19]$$

The basis that best separates the components is the one that best minimizes the covariance between the data and maximizes the variance term (Figure 4.9, left). Let us consider that the projection of the covariance matrix along a direction given by vector $\vec{u}$;$\vec{u}$ is the first vector of the PCA basis if this projection is maximal:

$$\begin{aligned} &\vec{u}, max(COV(\bar{M}) \cdot \vec{u}) \\ &\text{with} COV(\bar{M}) = \frac{1}{W}(\bar{M}^T \cdot \bar{M}) \end{aligned} \qquad [4.20]$$

In other terms, and following the Min-Max theorem, the consecutive vectors $\vec{u}$ are the eigenvectors of the covariance matrix. Eigenvectors follow:

$$(COV(\overline{M}) - \lambda I) \cdot \vec{u} = 0 \qquad [4.21]$$

The eigenvectors can be listed from the highest to the lowest eigenvalue, giving a transfer matrix denoted as $Ker(\overline{M})$. Then, each experiment $\vec{M}$, from the learning set or a new one, can be represented in the new basis after centering and reducing:

$$\vec{\breve{M}} = Ker(\overline{M})^T \vec{M} \qquad [4.22]$$

In the $Ker(\overline{M})$, the first eigenvectors have the higher influence (eigenvalue), and the last ones have the lower influence. The last eigenvectors mostly represent noise; thus, removing the last vectors is commonly used to remove noise. On the other way round, a question should be: what is the minimum number of vectors that adequately represent the phenomenon observed through the set of experiment M? If the eigenvectors are classified in a Pareto graph showing their influence on the total variance (Figure 4.9, right), it is possible to decide a threshold (usually set to 80% of the variance) and only keep the prominent terms. This approach can give drastic data reduction, for example, Chassagne et al. (2018) showed that only five parameters allow for representing any lower leg with an error smaller than 2 mm (Figure 4.10). This reduction was used later to define geometrical parameters in a meta-model.

In a more practical way, and denoting $K_{i,j}$ the kernel components:

$$\overrightarrow{M_{\text{Red}}} = \{ \begin{matrix} K^M_{1,1} & \cdots & K^M_{1,L_{\text{red}}<L} \\ \vdots & \ddots & \vdots \\ K^M_{N,1} & \cdots & K^M_{N,L_{\text{red}}<L} \end{matrix} \}^T \vec{M} \qquad [4.23]$$

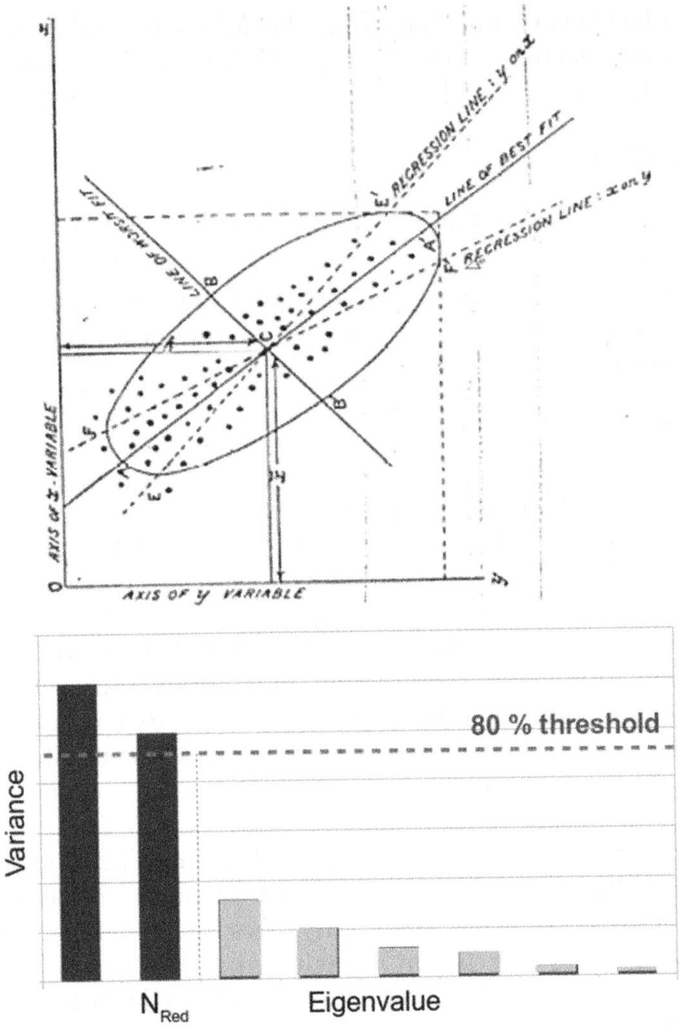

Figure 4.9. *Left: Representation of a data set on its natural basis and line of best and worst fit corresponding to the PCA basis from Pearson (1901). Right: rank of each independent variable in the output variance and model reduction (source: Chassagne et al. 2018). For a color version of this figure, see www.iste.co.uk/molimard/biomedicaldevices.zip*

Lastly, if the set of data is represented in only two dimensions (or at most 3), then PCA can help in classifying data[3]. For example, Bonnaire (2015) used PCA to classify lumbar belts and to discriminate relevant data in belt compression therapies (Figure 4.11).

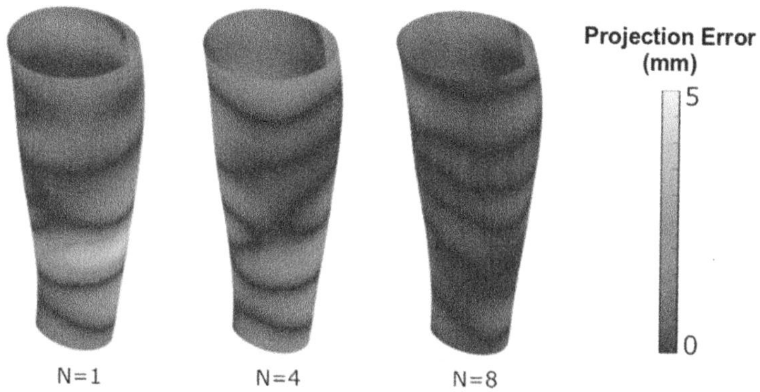

Figure 4.10. *Reconstruction of a leg on a PCA basis using a different number of vectors. If N ≥ 4, the error on the reconstruction is lower than 2 mm. Legs are normalized on their length (source: Chassagne et al. 2018). For a color version of this figure, see www.iste.co.uk/molimard/biomedicaldevices.zip*

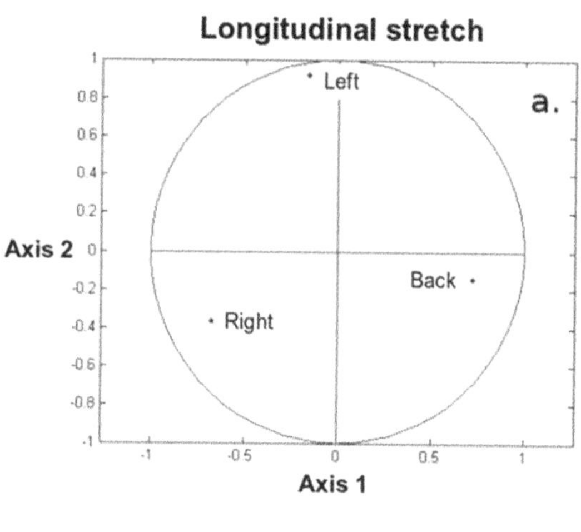

3 This feature is commonly used in text mining, but that is another story.

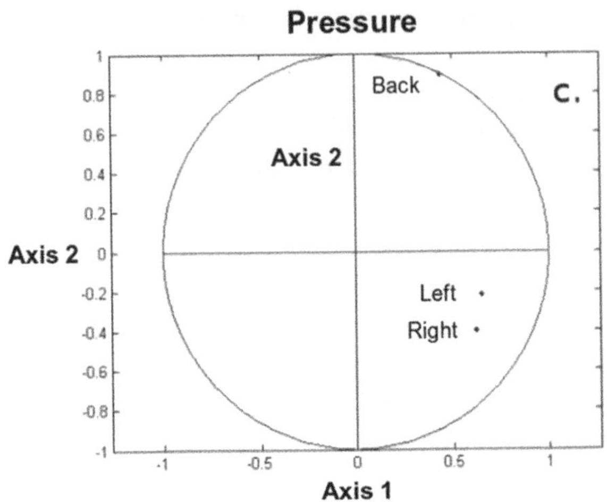

Figure 4.11. *PCA projection in 2D of longitudinal stretch in a lumbar belt and the corresponding pressure applied on the trunk for three locations (left, right and back). The charts show that left and right pressure are strongly correlated, but the stretches are independent (source: Bonnaire 2015). For a color version of this figure, see www.iste.co.uk/molimard/biomedicaldevices.zip*

4.2.5. *Exercises*

2D-video movement analysis

The purpose here is to follow the gait of a patient by using a smartphone-based application. The gait is videorecorded and the body is divided into segments with joints under rotation. A complete 3D solution has been presented in Pagnon et al. (2021); in this exercise, we propose to simplify to a 2D (one-camera) situation. Focal length f is supposed to be 30 mm.

Magnification is given by the size ratio between the real object (denoted AB) and its image counterpart ($A'B'$), following the equation (with d the distance between the camera lens and the object):

$$\frac{|AB|}{|A'B'|} = \frac{d}{f} \quad [4.24]$$

1) Nominal working distance d is 1.5 m. When walking or running, patients might move 0.3 m in the lateral direction. Using equation [4.24], extract the apparent size variation of the subject.

2) Propose a small Python or Octave program to describe the geometry of the leg (ankle, knee, hip) and to calculate the angle between thigh and lower leg considering that the leg (ankle-knee-hip) is on a plane. Note that it is obviously an incorrect hypothesis from the physiological point of view.

3) Let us suppose that the foot made a 0.3 m movement forward, the hip being at the same place. What would be the apparent angle at the knee level using a single camera?

4) Study the error with respect to the real angle and conclude on the quality of this measurement.

5) Assuming a normal statistical occurrence of the foot out of the image plane, express a global uncertainty range at 95% probability.

Force/strain measurement: effect of a temperature variation

A classical strain sensor is sensitive to mechanical strain, but in the case of temperature variation, the support dilates or contracts, giving a thermal strain that is not sought in most cases.

1) Considering a reasonable temperature variation of ±3°C, what would be the absolute uncertainty on strain measurement for a steel support and for a polymeric support?

2) We consider a set-up with an instrumented test body used under traction. To be conservative, the test body must be kept under the elastic regime, that is, below yield stress. Under a linear elastic hypothesis, what would be the yield strain for both materials? What is the relative uncertainty due to temperature changes in the two cases?

3) Considering previous results, what would you prescribe?

4) Find specific arrangements that could reduce the error related to thermal temperature in solid mechanics books (Molimard 2016) or online resources.

Material	Coef. of linear thermal expansion	Yield stress	Stiffness
Steel (X65)	$11.8 \times 10^{-6}\ K^{-1}$	448 MPa	210 GPa
Polypropylene	$150 \times 10^{-6}\ K^{-1}$	12 MPa	1.68 GPa

Table 4.3. *Error of the first and second kind*

5

Numerical Simulation and Medical Devices

5.1. Role of numerical simulation in medical device design

5.1.1. *General design workflow for medical device*

Figure 5.1 presents a general workflow for medical device design. This particular class of products is submitted to market approval. For the European Union, the supplier must prove that the medical device is safe for the patient; in the United States, the supplier must prove that the device is safe and efficient. The clinical trials are mandatory for the European Union and almost the same in the United States.

The design process is strongly influenced by the market approval requirements. No market approval can be given without a quality plan and without a post-market strategy (device follow-up).

In this context, the design validation can be based on cell engineering, small/large animal models or numerical modeling. In the following, numerical modeling, which is the cutting-edge technology in medical device development, will be explored in more detail.

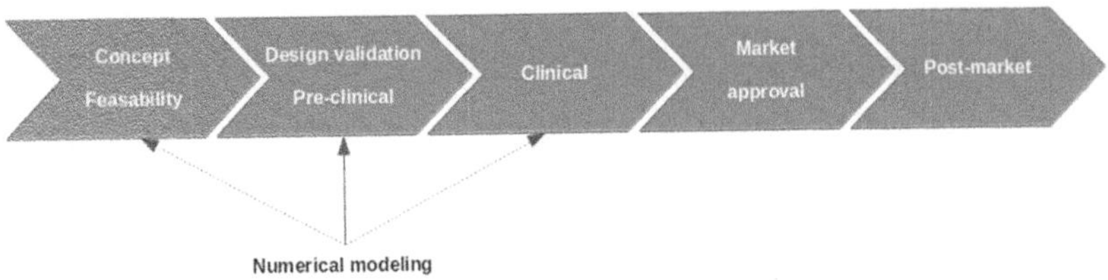

Figure 5.1. *General workflow for medical device and numerical modeling possible position*

5.1.2. *Introduction example*

Glaukos Corp designed a new intraocular pressure lowering implant (Nichamin 2009). It is composed of a stent and an injector. The stent is placed in the Schlemm canal and eases the fluid circulation between the anterior chamber and the blood vessels.

1) A finite element model was developed to check the structural integrity during the stent placement.

2) Key data in this work concern the pressure and flow characteristics in the Schlemm canal. Due to the difficulties in accessing these values through clinical trials (canal size, invasiveness of the measurement), a numerical model based on fluid dynamics has been used.

3) Lastly, MRI safety relies on the heating near a metallic part due to magnetic irradiation. This temperature rise can only be checked using multiphysics modeling. Here, the model concluded on a safe use on 3T or less MR systems if the exposure time is less than 15 min.

Among these three points, the first one is a basic mechanical engineer task. Other solutions (mechanical testing) could have led to a convenient result. Points 2 and 3 are more interesting: the data are difficult or impossible to measure experimentally, even if they are driven factors in the claimed effect.

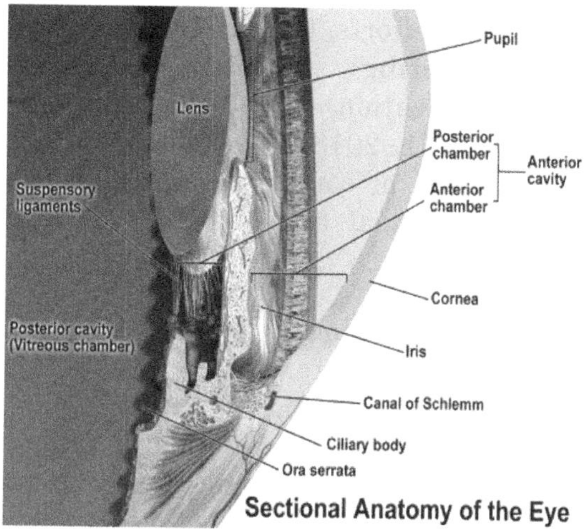

Figure 5.2. *Eye description. Canal of Schlemm links the anterior chamber to episcleral blood vessels (Blausen Medical 2014). For a color version of this figure, see www.iste.co.uk/molimard/biomedicaldevices.zip*

5.2. General context

5.2.1. *Agency policies*

Even if numerical modeling has been used for years in medical devices, the FDA published its first document on computational modeling studies in medical devices in 2014, and this became a reference two years later (FDA 2016). This document provides recommendations to support medical device submissions. In some cases, a full numerical modeling process can be used for product submission.

Numerical modeling could be used in many fields of physics: solid mechanics (e.g. ultrasounds, articular prosthesis, stent and hospital bedrest), fluid mechanics (e.g. extra-corporal blood circulation and lab-on-chip devices), electromagnetism (magnetic resonance imaging), optics (e.g. endoscopic devices) and thermal propagation (e.g. high-intensity focused ultrasound).

Besides the FDA's efforts, the ASME (American Society of Mechanical Engineering) recently published its 3rd validation and verification (V&V) document dedicated to medical devices (ASME 2018). V&V documents report good practices on the V&V of computational modeling in solids (V&V 10), fluids and heat transfer (V&V 20) and recently medical devices (V&V 40).

In the European Union, the new Medical Devices Regulation (2017/745/EU) reinforces the role of clinical evidence[1]. Numerical modeling enters in the preclinical evaluation process as well as the bibliography and results on animal models. No recommendation has been published to date.

Besides these regulatory or normative aspects, the Committee on Credible Practice of Modeling and Simulation in Healthcare (Erdemir et al. 2020) has proposed a set of rules beyond the well-admitted verification and validation approach. They are listed as follows:

1) Define context clearly.

2) Use contextually appropriate data.

3) Evaluate within context.

4) List limitations explicitly.

5) Use version control.

6) Document appropriately.

7) Disseminate broadly.

8) Obtain independent reviews.

9) Test competing implementations.

10) Conform to standards.

---

1 See: https://ec.europa.eu/growth/single-market/european-standards/harmonised-standards/medical-devices_en.

Most of these quality rules are already known in the engineering community, but the authors stress the necessity to recall them, as they are poorly followed. The ASME and FDA recommendations, even if they could not explicitly refer to these rules that have been published later, respect them in practice.

5.2.2. *Report structure*

Although being close and compatible, the report structures recommended by the ASME and FDA are slightly different. Table 5.1 shows the global framework of each.

A first difference is in the place where the system (MD) is described. The FDA exposes the description after the code description, whereas the ASME includes it in the background. But the main differences lie in the ASME complementary contribution. First, the context of use (COU) defines the question the numerical model is built for. This point is implicit in the FDA approach but putting it forward as in the former gives the report a structure closer to clinical testing. For engineers, the choices in designing a numerical model strongly depend on the question to address. Clarifying this is a clue in the confidence for this model.

Second, the AMSE proposal is based on V&V. It focuses on the model validation *regarding a risk factor*. Of course, the efforts to put in the numerical model will depend on the consequences of the decisions that will result from it.

A summary is proposed in Table 5.1. Of course, a brief summary has to be given, as well as references. These points do not need too much of an explanation; the other points will be developed below.

Synthesis	FDA recommendations	ASME V&V 40
(1) Executive report summary	(1) Executive report summary	
(2) Background	(2) Background/introduction (4) System configuration (6) System properties	(1) Background Device Process System Clinical application
(3) Question of interest		(2) Context of use of the computational model
(4) Computation model	(3) Code verification (5) Governing equations/constitutive laws (7) System conditions (8) System discretization (9) Numerical implementation	(3) Computational model details
(5) Model risk		(4) Model risk Model influence Decision consequence
(6) Model validation	(10) Validation	(5) Credibility activities Verification Validation Applicability of the validation activities to the COU
(7) Results	(11) Results	(5bis) Results
(8) Computational model credibility assessment	(12) Discussion (13) Limitations	(5ter) Computational model credibility assessment
(9) Conclusions	(14) Conclusions	
(10) References	(15) References	

Table 5.1. *Comparison of report structure as recommended by FDA2018 and ASME2018 V&V40*

5.3. Report details

5.3.1. *Background*

The background should detail the device and its correlative instrument set, as well as give information that helps the reader to understand the technical question addressed and the numerical model. In addition, it is important to give an overview of the role of the numerical study in the medical device development.

5.3.2. *Question of interest*

The question of interest for the numerical study is the scientific or technical question to address. It should be expressed as a clinical question, with a dual true/false answer. Other indications (e.g. coming from clinical study and bibliography) should delimit the scope of the question.

Here, a small description on the strategy developed to answer this question (context of use) must be detailed. This description should give an indication for the numerical model[2] to use it in a proper way.

EXAMPLE.–

Medical device: Lumbar belt

---

2 Formally, the context of use is "the actual conditions under which a given artifact/software product is used or will be used in a normal day to day working situation. It is important to carry out usability tests, prototyping sessions, meetings, user studies and other 'user-dependent sessions' in the context of use to get as high ecological validity (see this) of your findings as possible", as defined by the Interaction Design Foundation, The Glossary of Human Computer Interaction, available at: https://www.interaction-design.org/literature/book/the-glossary-of-human-computer-interaction/context-of-use.

Question of interest: does the lumbar belt relieve pain for the patients?

Context of use: following usual belt manufacturer claims, we make the hypothesis that the lumbar belt has a mechanical effect on the body in the short term. Even if the literature shows that the orign of pain is much more complicated than this, we will focus only on the delordosing effect of the belt. A numerical model is designed to describe the pressure applied by the MD on the body, and it gives a quantitative indicator of delordosing. The belt will be designed on a numerical interface. Its mechanical properties will be calculated using the mechanical properties of each individual component, as given in the suppliers' technical datasheets. The numerical model will take advantage of real patient trunk shapes and should adapt to different kinds of morphology, in particular by adjusting the belt size (Molimard et al. 2019).

5.3.3. *Computation model*

This section reinforces the confidence on the study and its conclusions. It shows how good practices have been respected. This section describes the tools and assumptions.

Software quality assurance: in many cases, the study is based on finite element modeling or computational fluid dynamics. Of course, a commercial software, with a high level of verification, would give a better credibility than a home-made code, freeware mostly lying in between. In the case of the home-made code, the V&V process should be detailed more. Code verification activities are recommended even for commercial software and comparing numerical results to benchmark (analytical) solutions is the most common method. The FDA (2002) particularly outlines the role of management and quality process throughout the software development as part of the quality assurance.

The "model" in itself, that is, the part geometry, the boundary conditions, constitutive equations and the discretization used, is of course the more important part.

Model form: continuum physics phenomena (solid or fluid mechanics: thermal transfer, electromagnetism, etc.) are described by a differential equation that links physics quantities and/or their derivatives (see example below). This equation is based on the assumptions on the phenomena occurring that may be linked together or not. For example, is the blood flow (*fluid mechanics*) in a cancerous skin tumor also dependent on the temperature (*thermal transfer*)?

Constitutive laws: each physics equation depends on the way the material reacts to a solicitation. In mechanics, it could be elastic (linear or not), viscous (Newtonian or not), plastic, isotropic or anisotropic, etc. The R&D engineer must choose these constitutive laws and fill them with values. The properties associated with the system to be studied correspond both to the medical device but also to the human body. Human body properties are always difficult to find, contradictory from one author to the other. In short terms, it is necessary to give as much information as possible to increase the quality of the study.

Boundary conditions: another property of this equation is that it is valid for any infinitesimal piece of material inside the medium. To solve this equation, we need to use boundary conditions and initial conditions (if time is a parameter). The boundary conditions are in most cases a key point in mechanical validation and should be considered very carefully.

Solving parameters: this equation can be solved in many ways; a popular one consists of splitting the volume into elements and finding an approximate solution on these little elements. The solution has a certain shape, usually a linear or quadratic function and minimize the energy error. This finite elements method needs the user to choose the shape, function and the size of the elements. Of course, these choices must be verified: does the result depend on the size of the elements (convergence analysis)? Is the result stable with the time step?

Geometrical modeling: another question to make explicit is the definition of the geometry. In classical engineering, this consists mainly of choosing the level of details we would put in the model. The more details that are kept, the bigger the memory necessary for the problem and the longer the processing time will be. In medical engineering, the description of the organ is much more difficult and depends on each patient and on the imaging technique used. This leads to a functional compromise that is at the core of engineering: simplifications make the problem have a solution, but the interpretation of the results cannot exceed the limitations given by aforementioned simplifications.

Quantification of sensitivities: the more all of these choices are explained and justified, the higher the confidence of the numerical model results will be. In addition, it is possible for most of the previous elements to perform a sensitivity analysis giving a *budget*[3] on the results, for example:

– variation in the maximum stress in a structure depending on the element size;

– variation in the pressure in a vessel regarding its stiffness range (that should be associated with authors, methodology or subject intervariability);

---

3 An uncertainty budget is a table of components that contribute to the uncertainty in measurement results. It identifies, quantifies and characterizes each independent variable. With respect to measurement quality, it is an essential tool to perform uncertainty analysis. See, for example, https://www.muelaner.com/uncertainty-of-measurement/.

– effect of measured quantity (e.g. geometry of a vessel) on a derived (calculated) quantity (e.g. the corresponding pressure).

EXAMPLE.–

The heat equation is one of the simpler equations. It concerns the conservation of energy, that is here, the equilibrium between the heat flow and the temperature rate:

$$\frac{\partial u}{\partial t} = \frac{k}{C.\rho}\left(\frac{\partial^2 u}{\partial x^2} + \frac{\partial^2 u}{\partial y^2} + \frac{\partial^2 u}{\partial z^2}\right)$$

where c is the specific heat capacity, ρ is the density and k is the thermal conductivity.

Boundary conditions: on contour Γ_1, $u(t, x \in \Gamma_1) = U_{\Gamma_1}$

on contour Γ_2, $\frac{\partial u(t,x \in \Gamma_2)}{\partial n} = \Phi_{\Gamma_2}$

(n: direction normal to the surface)

Initial condition: $\forall x \in \Omega, u(0,x) = u_{init}(x)$

5.3.4. *Model risk*

The risk associated with the model is the risk it presents for the user. The risk range is very wide, from time delay to harm (or even handicap or death). For example, constant sliding on the thigh because of a knee brace design failure would lead to skin injuries. Removing the knee brace for a while would make the skin recover quickly. In this case, the error in the model that leads to a wrong design has a moderate influence and the risk level is moderate (considering that giving up the treatment would have consequences on the recovery). If the sliding now occurs inside an artery between a stent graft and the artery, there is no possibility to stop the injury that could degrade the artery wall and the consequences would be more serious, for example, revision surgery.

Of course, the risk has to be mitigated considering the importance of the model in the decision. If the model is the only way to decide a risky choice, its importance is higher. Often, this is not the case and the numerical model is only a component in decision-making that is used to design clinical tests.

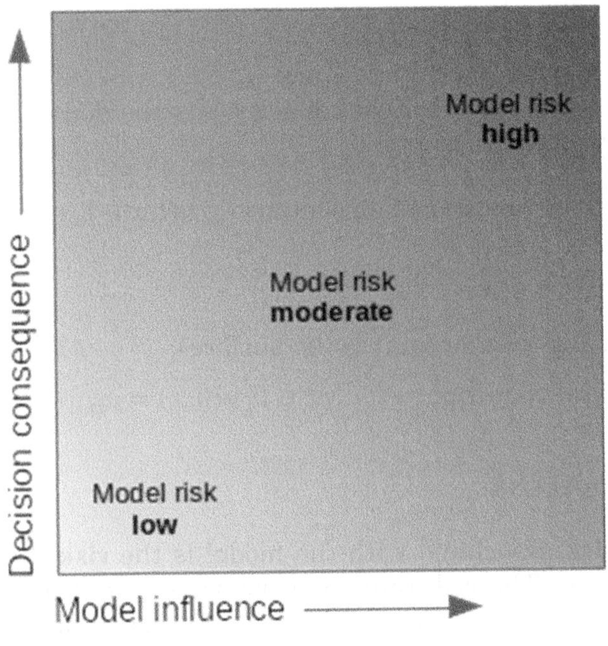

Figure 5.3. *Components of the model risk (qualitative representation). For a color version of this figure, see www.iste.co.uk/molimard/biomedicaldevices.zip*

Finally, the importance of the numerical model is a combination of the decision consequence and the model influence (Figure 5.3).

Designers should decide and give a ranking for both the model influence (from *minor fact on the decision* to *significant*) and the decision consequence (from *minor impact on the patient* to *severe patient injuries or death*).

5.3.5. *Model validation*

Validation of a model is much more than verifying the code, as it is expected in the section on the computation model. It aims to evaluate how far the numerical model is from reality, and therefore discusses the validity of the geometrical simplifications, boundary conditions, physics or material assumptions, etc. Model validation needs a reference. The degree of complexity of the reference could vary with the application. This could be a reference model, an analytical solution or an experimental set of results (from the lab, taken from literature, from clinics).

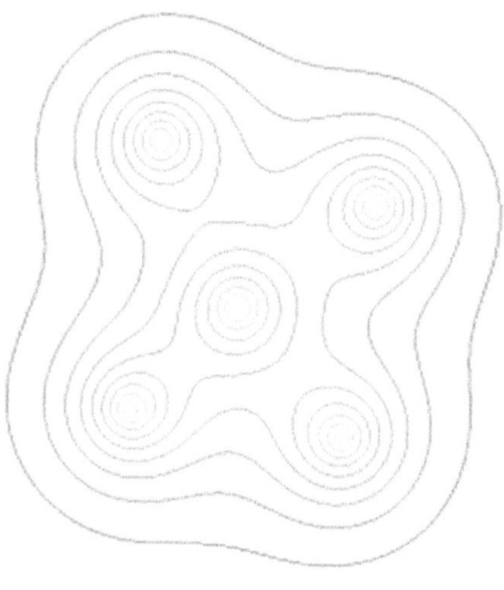

Figure 5.4. *2D symbolic representation of the model credibility after verification on five situations. For a color version of this figure, see www.iste.co.uk/molimard/biomedicaldevices.zip*

The quality of the reference (bias and random error in measuring process, etc.) is crucial in the validation process and will limit the conclusion. For example, an in vitro test-bench should be used with reference material rather than a real biological sample in order to reduce reference variability. This would imply that this reference material is correctly defined: silicon-based material is commonly used to represent a soft tissue; an elastic assumption is only correct in a certain range in time and stress or strain. Then a convenient comparison is possible but the domain of the model is wider and this validation can be improved by mapping the domain of the model. The confidence to the model then depends on the number of validation points the designers should provide (see Figure 5.4).

5.3.6. *Ranking the model credibility*

The ASME V&V40 recommends to evaluate the quality of the overall procedure by ranking both verification and validation steps. Giving a clear description on the quality levels and what has been achieved is part of the discussion with the designers' partners (banks, medical agencies, etc.). Ranking should be provided for each activity.

EXAMPLE: SOFTWARE QUALITY ASSURANCE (SQA).–

Graduation proposed by the ASME would reflect the rigor on the software SQA:

a) Very little or no SQA procedure.

b) SQA procedures specified and documented.

c) SQA procedures specified and documented; the software anomaly list is well understood and its consequence on the conditions of use is discussed; quality metrics are tracked.

EXAMPLE: USER ERRORS.–

The main error source in some cases should be the user itself, and the way the software is organized:

a) Inputs and outputs are not verified.

b) Inputs and outputs are verified by users and internal peer reviewer.

c) Inputs and outputs are verified by reproducing simulation by external peer reviewer.

EXAMPLE: OUTPUT COMPARISON IN VALIDATION TASKS (ADAPTED FROM ASME V&V40).–

The aim is to scale the rigor in the comparison between numerical model and external reference.

a) Visual comparison.

b) Comparison by measuring the difference between the two sets of results: differences ≤ 20%.

c) Comparison by measuring the difference between the two sets of results: differences ≤ 10%.

d) Comparison by measuring the difference between the two sets of results: differences ≤ 10%.

Uncertainties are estimated and provided.

e) Comparison by measuring the difference between the two sets of results: differences ≤ 10%.

Uncertainties are estimated and provided: rigorous statistical testing on the difference is provided.

5.3.7. *Computational model credibility assessment*

Credibility assessment should be considered as a fundamental senior engineering task, as it is based on good practice and experience. In any case, some basic methodologies, derived from clinical testing, can be used in order to increase the computational model credibility:

1) As stated before, this activity should be performed by well-trained professionals.

2) Credibility criteria should be stated *before* going to modeling tasks (both verification and results production). In this way, the influence on the actual results is limited.

3) Results of the computational model credibility assessment should be reviewed by people – inside or outside the company – not involved in the project that would not understand its objectives and challenges.

The results of the credibility assessments may not comply with the criteria: in case of a test fail, a discussion should be developed in order to map the effect of the given validation failure on future results. This may (1) reduce the validity domain – and remove some COU from the target list – but may be considered as sufficient; (2) lead to the inclusion of extra features to the computational model (in this case, note that the decision would require a new validation round); (3) decrease the influence of the computational model by adding extra information from other numerical models, experimental work, etc.; (4) prompt the designers to change their strategy and go for experimental or clinical works.

5.3.8. *Results and discussion*

The results section should carefully recall the Question of Interest, the model limitations and results, both in graphical and table formats. The discussion should recall the credibility assessment work, but it has to go further by comparing the numerical results with the other experimental or clinical studies and the state-of-the-art literature. Results obtained for a new device should be compared to other devices already in use, and in particular to the gold standard.

PERSONAL PRACTICE.– Read and analyze the publication:

> Aldieri, A., Curreli, C., Szyszko, J.A., La Mattina, A.A., Viceconti, M. (2023). Credibility

assessment of computational models according to ASME V&V40: Application to the Bologna Biomechanical Computed Tomography solution. *Computer Methods and Programs in Biomedicine*, 240, 107727. doi: 10.1016/j.cmpb.2023.107727.

1) Identify the seven steps defined above.

2) To what extent does the work cover the 10 items identified by the Committee on Credible Practice of Modeling and Simulation in Healthcare?

6

Global Ethics Rule Beyond Clinical Trials

6.1. Medical ethics, from Hippocrates to the Declaration of Geneva

Medical ethics has a long history, mixing corporate rules, religion and science. One of the oldest texts relating to medical ethics is the Hippocratic Oath. Even though Hippocrates lived ca. 460–370 BCE, the oldest manuscript fragment dates to ca. 275 CE. A lot of interpretations of the text have arisen, as it has to be established in a certain historical and societal background and the latter is seen in another historical and societal context. May we consider the following here:

– The oath is made before gods and goddesses (Apollo, Asclepius, Hygieia and Panacea). This has been modified later as religion changed (God, even "Supreme Being" during the French revolution!), but the role of religion in medical ethics, as well as representations of illness and healing, is obvious before the Enlightenment, especially with the rise of monotheic religions in the Roman and Greek world.

– The medical knowledge should be kept within the medical community.

– The use of the scalpel is discarded. This should initiate the historical difference between physicians and surgeons. An interpretation is that a doctor should not go beyond their competence.

– Medical knowledge is prohibited to be used against life (*Primum non nocere*, even if the phrase has been introduced later). The oath proscribes the use of poison, euthanasia or even abortion – maybe infanticide, depending again on the interpretation.

– The medical confidentiality is stated.

Despite its prestige, the Hippocratic Oath was not respected in the Roman world, as medicine was not regulated. A lot of doctors practiced euthanasia, in particular, under Imperial orders. The arrival of Judeo-Christian morality has disrupted this situation. During the third to fourth century, Assaph Ha-Yehoudi, a doctor from Syria, encouraged the care for the poor people free of charge. Later, Ishaq ibn'Ali al-Ruhawi wrote *Adab al-Tabib* (Physician's practical morality), where he presented the doctor as a mediator between the patient and God. For him, becoming a doctor required a virtuous predisposition (pious, sensitive, literate and temperate). In the medieval Occident, medicine slowly became a liberal art, and surgery a manual art taught in the universities, for example, Montpellier School of Medicine funded during the 13th century, nowadays the oldest school of medicine in the world[1], and adapted forms of the Hippocratic Oath were used. One of the last great texts on medical ethics before the Modern age was the *Maimonides' medical prayer* (written in 1783), but referring to Moses ben

1 The Schola Medica Salernitana, funded during the 9th century, is probably the most important school of medicine of the Middle Ages. It disseminated in the Western world the antique, Byzantine and Arabic medicines. It became a university during the 13th century but disappeared during the 14th century.

Maimon (known as Maimonides), a physician of the 12th century born in Spain and who died in Egypt. The prayer develops the theme of medical knowledge: the physician must consider the limits of their knowledge in their care; they always have the will to learn. Similarly, they have to defend their patient from charlatans.

The medicine of the Enlightenment, refunded by the anatomo-clinical method and experimental physiology, was not well adapted to the Hippocratic heritage. Even if his moral legacy is not called into question, modern notions of ethics and deontology pushed Thomas Percival (England) to write a modern code of medical ethics. In 1803, he published "Medical Ethics, or a Code of Institutes and Precepts, Adapted to the Professional Conduct of Physicians and Surgeons". This code would have a great influence in English-speaking countries. Since its adoption in 1847, it has been periodically revised in the United States. In France, Dr. Simon carried out a similar work in 1845's "Déontologie médicale ou des devoirs et des droits des médecins dans l'état actuel de la civilisation", but its impact would be more limited. For many years during the 19th century, the medical doctors organized to defend their interest in the College of Physicians and deontology; rules were made to foster exchange between practitioners.

In modern times, the Hippocratic Oath is a symbolic gateway for a student to become a professional in many countries. Its modern form is the Declaration of Geneva, although many countries still use the Hippocratic Oath with some variation.

DECLARATION OF GENEVA (IN ITS ACTUAL FORM).–

As a member of the medical profession:

– I solemnly pledge to dedicate my life to the service of humanity.

– The health and well-being of my patient will be my first consideration.

– I will respect the autonomy and dignity of my patient.

– I will maintain the utmost respect for human life.

– I will not permit considerations of age, disease or disability, creed, ethnic origin, gender, nationality, political affiliation, race, sexual orientation, social standing or any other factor to intervene between my duty and my patient.

– I will respect the secrets that are confided in me, even after the patient has died.

– I will practice my profession with conscience and dignity and in accordance with good medical practice.

– I will foster the honor and noble traditions of the medical profession.

– I will give to my teachers, colleagues and students the respect and gratitude that is their due.

– I will share my medical knowledge for the benefit of the patient and the advancement of healthcare.

– I will attend to my own health, well-being and abilities in order to provide care of the highest standard.

– I will not use my medical knowledge to violate human rights and civil liberties, even under threat.

– I make these promises solemnly, freely and upon my honor.

6.2. Evolution of ethics rules for clinical trials

At the end of World War II, the allies discovered the horror of tests on humans performed by Nazi physicians. During the Nuremberg trials, the Doctors' Trial brought to light that no formal text stated what would be an acceptable or an unacceptable clinical test. The Court mandated for two experts to give a state of the art review on clinical practice. In 1947, Dr L. Alexander and Pr A. Ivy drew up a list of 10 criteria known as the Nuremberg Code, defining what are Permissible Medical Experiments. The year 1947 became a turning point in clinical research.

In reality, few attempts were made before 1947. We can mention C. Bernard[2], the founder of experimental medicine, who wrote in 1856 “Among the experiments that can be tried on humans, those that can only harm are forbidden, those that are innocent are allowed, and those that can do good are recommended” (Bernard 1856). Ironically, it turns out that Germany had the most advanced code just before the Nazis came to power. In 1931, a ministerial circular, the Reichsrundschreiben, provided a framework for human medical experimentation. The aim was to protect subjects and patients, while encouraging research. Its principles were the individual responsibility of researchers, the search for minimum risk, absolute respect for children, the weak and the dying, and above all the “unequivocal” and “unambiguous” consent of patients or subjects of the experiment.

In western democracies, the Nuremberg Code had not been considered as useful in the normal situations of democratic countries but only as a text for exceptional situations; and questionable experiments were carried out without proper control or ethics guidelines (e.g. Tuskegee Syphilis Study, Operation Whitecoat in the United States, Vipeholm experiments in Sweden and many others). However, the Nuremberg Code turned out to be a very important contribution to ethics and gave rise in 1964 to the universal Declaration of Helsinki, promoted by the World Medical Association (WMA). Both the Nuremberg Code and Declaration of Helsinki are references used in the present

2 Lyon used the name “Claude Bernard” for the university of Physics and Medicine, in tribute to one of its most outstanding citizens.

day in the institutional review board. This has inspired legal texts in the United States (Electronic Code of Federal Regulations, title 45, part 46 "Protection of Human subjects"[3]) and in Europe (Directive 2001/83/EC, on the Community code relating to medicinal products for human use[4] and Directive 2001/20/EC, on the approximation of the laws, regulations and administrative provisions of the Member States relating to the implementation of good clinical practice in the conduct of clinical trials on medicinal products for human use[5]) and the standard ISO14155 "Clinical investigation of medical devices for human subjects-Good Clinical Practice"[6].

Another good clinical practice standard is provided by the International Conference on Harmonisation of Technical Requirements for Registration of Pharmaceuticals for Human Use (ICH 1995). The ICH-GCP is recognized by both the EU and the United States agencies as reference rules. However, even though the organization explicitly refers to the Declaration of Helsinki, criticisms came out and the ICH-GCP is considered to be less ethical and more procedural than its predecessor. In particular, the decision-making is only based on representatives of three agencies (the United States, EU and Japan), instead of plenary sessions of the Council for International Organizations of Medical Sciences; the ICH-GCP guidelines do not address conflict of interest, the need to publish results, or post-trial availability of

3 Electronic Code of Federal Regulations: https://www.ecfr.gov/cgi-bin/textidx?SID=4720e94ab56747f24940d77ced30e838&mc=true&node=pt45.1.46&rgn=div5 (14 November 2019).

4 DIRECTIVE 2001/83/EC OF THE EUROPEAN PARLIAMENT AND OF THE COUNCIL of November 6, 2001: https://eur-lex.europa.eu/legal-content/EN/TXT/?uri=CELEX%3A02001L0083-20220101.

5 DIRECTIVE 2001/20/EC OF THE EUROPEAN PARLIAMENT AND OF THE COUNCIL of April 4, 2001: https://eur-lex.europa.eu/legal-content/EN/ALL/?uri=CELEX:02001L0020-20090807.

6 Available at: http://www.imdrf.org/docs/imdrf/final/meetings/imdrf-meet-160913-brazil-iso14155-2011.pdf or https://www.iso.org/standard/71690.html.

successful treatments to study participants or community members (Lurie and Greco 2005). Nevertheless, the Declaration of Helsinki is the only ethics framework recognized by International Committee of Medical Journal Editors[7], which reads "All investigators should ensure that the planning conduct and reporting of human research are in accordance with the Helsinki Declaration as revised in 2013".

THE 10 POINTS OF THE NUREMBERG CODE.–

– The voluntary consent of the human subject is absolutely essential.

– The experiment should be such as to yield fruitful results for the good of society, unprocurable by other methods or means of study, and not random and unnecessary in nature.

– The experiment should be so designed and based on the results of animal experimentation and a knowledge of the natural history of the disease or other problems under study that the anticipated results will justify the performance of the experiment.

– The experiment should be so conducted as to avoid all unnecessary physical and mental suffering and injury.

– No experiment should be conducted where there is an a priori reason to believe that death or disabling injury will occur; except, perhaps, in those experiments where the experimental physicians also serve as subjects.

– The degree of risk to be taken should never exceed that determined by the humanitarian importance of the problem to be solved by the experiment.

7 ICMJE gathers 13 journals, including: *The Lancet*, *JAMA*, *New England Journal of Medicine*. Hundreds of journals refer to ICMJE for their publication rules.

– Proper preparations should be made and adequate facilities provided to protect the experimental subject against even remote possibilities of injury, disability or death.

– The experiment should be conducted only by scientifically qualified persons. The highest degree of skill and care should be required through all stages of the experiment of those who conduct (or engage) in the experiment.

– During the course of the experiment, the human subject should be at liberty to bring the experiment to an end if they have reached the physical or mental state where continuation of the experiment seems to them to be impossible.

– During the course of the experiment, the scientist in charge must be prepared to terminate the experiment at any stage, if they have probable cause to believe, in the exercise of the good faith, superior skill and careful judgment required of them, that a continuation of the experiment is likely to result in injury, disability or death to the experimental subject.

6.3. Declaration of Helsinki

The Declaration of Helsinki is mentioned below. Even though point 1 states that the Declaration is intended to be read as a whole, some key notions are outlined in this reprint – but not in the original production.

Preamble

1) The World Medical Association (WMA) has developed the Declaration of Helsinki as a statement of ethical principles for medical research involving human subjects, including research on identifiable human material and data.

The Declaration is intended to be read as a whole and each of its constituent paragraphs should be applied with consideration of all other relevant paragraphs.

2) Consistent with the mandate of the WMA, *the Declaration is addressed primarily to physicians. The WMA encourages others who are involved in medical research involving human subjects to adopt these principles.*

General principles

3) The Declaration of Geneva of the WMA binds the physician with the words, "The health of my patient will be my first consideration", and the International Code of Medical Ethics declares that, "A physician shall act in the patient's best interest when providing medical care".

4) It is the *duty of the physician to promote and safeguard the health, well-being and rights of patients*, including those who are involved in medical research. The physician's knowledge and conscience are dedicated to the fulfillment of this duty.

5) Medical progress is based on research that ultimately must include studies involving human subjects.

6) The primary purpose of medical research involving human subjects is to understand the causes, development and effects of diseases and improve preventive, diagnostic and therapeutic interventions (methods, procedures and treatments). Even the best proven interventions must be evaluated continually through research for their safety, effectiveness, efficiency, accessibility and quality.

7) Medical research is subject to ethical standards that promote and ensure respect for all human subjects and protect their health and rights.

8) *While the primary purpose of medical research is to generate new knowledge, this goal can never take precedence over the rights and interests of individual research subjects.*

9) It is the *duty of physicians who are involved in medical research to protect the life, health, dignity, integrity, right to self-determination, privacy and confidentiality of personal information of research subjects.* The responsibility for the protection of research subjects must always rest with the physician or other health care professionals and never with the research subjects, even though they have given consent.

10) Physicians must consider the ethical, legal and regulatory norms and standards for research involving human subjects in their own countries as well as applicable international norms and standards. *No national or international ethical, legal or regulatory requirement should reduce or eliminate any of the protections for research subjects set forth in this Declaration.*

11) Medical research should be conducted in a manner that minimizes possible harm to the environment.

12) *Medical research involving human subjects must be conducted only by individuals with the appropriate ethics and scientific education, training and qualifications.* Research on patients or healthy volunteers requires the supervision of a competent and appropriately qualified physician or other healthcare professional.

13) Groups that are underrepresented in medical research should be provided appropriate access to participation in research.

14) Physicians who combine medical research with medical care should involve their patients in research only to the extent that this is justified by its potential preventive, diagnostic or therapeutic value, and if the physician has good

reason to believe that participation in the research study will not adversely affect the health of the patients who serve as research subjects.

15) *Appropriate compensation and treatment* for subjects who are harmed as a result of participating in research must be ensured.

Risks, burdens and benefits

16) In medical practice and in medical research, most interventions involve risks and burdens.

Medical research involving human subjects may only be conducted if the importance of the objective outweighs the risks and burdens to the research subjects.

17) *All medical research involving human subjects must be preceded by careful assessment of predictable risks and burdens* to the individuals and groups involved in the research in comparison with foreseeable benefits to them and to other individuals (or groups) affected by the condition under investigation.

Measures to minimize the risks must be implemented. *The risks must be continuously monitored, assessed and documented by the researcher.*

18) Physicians may not be involved in a research study involving human subjects, unless they are confident that the risks have been adequately assessed and can be satisfactorily managed.

When the risks are found to outweigh the potential benefits or when there is conclusive proof of definitive outcomes, physicians must assess whether to continue, modify or immediately stop the study.

Vulnerable groups and individuals

19) Some groups and individuals are particularly vulnerable and may have an increased likelihood of being wronged or of incurring additional harm.

All vulnerable groups and individuals should receive specifically considered protection.

20) Medical research with a vulnerable group is only justified if the research is responsive to the health needs or priorities of this group and the research cannot be carried out in a non-vulnerable group. In addition, this group should stand to benefit from the knowledge, practices or interventions that result from the research.

Scientific requirements and research protocols

21) *Medical research involving human subjects must conform to generally accepted scientific principles, be based on a thorough knowledge of the scientific literature*, other relevant sources of information, and an adequate laboratory; and, as appropriate, animal experimentation. The welfare of animals used for research must be respected.

22) *The design and performance of each research study involving human subjects must be clearly described and justified in a research protocol.*

The protocol should contain a statement of the ethical considerations involved and should indicate how the principles in this Declaration have been addressed. *The protocol should include information regarding funding, sponsors, institutional affiliations, potential conflicts of interest, incentives for subjects and information regarding provisions for treating and/or compensating subjects who are harmed as a consequence of participation in the research study.*

In clinical trials, the protocol must also describe appropriate arrangements for post-trial provisions.

Research ethics committees

23) *The research protocol must be submitted for consideration, comment, guidance and approval to the concerned research ethics committee before the study begins.* This committee must be transparent in its functioning, must be independent of the researcher, the sponsor and any other undue influence, and must be duly qualified. It must take into consideration the laws and regulations of the country or countries in which the research is to be performed as well as applicable international norms and standards; however, these must not be allowed to reduce or eliminate any of the protections for research subjects set forth in this Declaration.

The committee must have the right to monitor ongoing studies. *The researcher must provide monitoring information to the committee, especially information about any serious adverse events.* No amendment to the protocol may be made without consideration and approval by the committee. *After the end of the study, the researchers must submit a final report to the committee* containing a summary of the study's findings and conclusions.

Privacy and confidentiality

24) Every precaution must be taken to *protect the privacy of research subjects* and the confidentiality of their personal information.

Informed consent

25) Participation by individuals capable of giving informed consent as subjects in medical research must be

voluntary. Although it may be appropriate to consult family members or community leaders, *no individual capable of giving informed consent may be enrolled in a research study unless they freely agree.*

26) In medical research involving human subjects capable of giving informed consent, *each potential subject must be adequately informed* of the aims, methods, sources of funding, any possible conflicts of interest, institutional affiliations of the researcher, the anticipated benefits and potential risks of the study and the discomfort it may entail, post-study provisions and any other relevant aspects of the study. The potential subject must be informed of the right to refuse to participate in the study or to withdraw consent to participate at any time without reprisal. Special attention should be given to the specific information needs of individual potential subjects as well as to the methods used to deliver the information.

After ensuring that the potential subject has understood the information, *the physician* or another appropriately qualified individual *must then seek the potential subject's freely given informed consent, preferably in writing.* If the consent cannot be expressed in writing, the non-written consent must be formally documented and witnessed.

All medical research subjects should be given the option of being informed about the general outcome and results of the study.

27) When seeking informed consent for participation in a research study, the physician must be particularly cautious if the potential subject is in a dependent relationship with the physician or may consent under duress. In such situations, the informed consent must be sought by an appropriately qualified individual who is completely independent of this relationship.

28) For a potential research subject who is incapable of giving informed consent, the physician must seek informed consent from the legally authorized representative. These individuals must not be included in a research study that has no likelihood of benefit for them, unless it is intended to promote the health of the group represented by the potential subject, the research cannot instead be performed with persons capable of providing informed consent, and the research entails only minimal risk and minimal burden.

29) When a potential research subject who is deemed incapable of giving informed consent is able to give assent to decisions about participation in research, the physician must seek that assent in addition to the consent of the legally authorized representative. The potential subject's dissent should be respected.

30) Research involving subjects who are physically or mentally incapable of giving consent (for example, unconscious patients) may be done only if the physical or mental condition that prevents giving informed consent is a necessary characteristic of the research group. In such circumstances, the physician must seek informed consent from the legally authorized representative. If no such representative is available and if the research cannot be delayed, the study may proceed without informed consent, provided that the specific reasons for involving subjects with a condition that renders them unable to give informed consent have been stated in the research protocol and the study has been approved by a research ethics committee. Consent to remain in the research must be obtained as soon as possible from the subject or a legally authorized representative.

31) The physician must fully inform the patient which aspects of their care are related to the research. *The refusal of a patient to participate in a study or the patient's decision to withdraw from the study must never adversely affect the patient–physician relationship.*

32) For medical research using identifiable human material or data, such as research on material or data contained in biobanks or similar repositories, physicians must seek informed consent for its collection, storage and/or reuse. There may be exceptional situations where consent would be impossible or impracticable to obtain for such research. In such situations, the research may be done only after consideration and approval of a research ethics committee.

Use of placebo

33) The benefits, risks, burdens and effectiveness of *a new intervention must be tested against those of the best proven intervention(s)*, except in the following circumstances:

Where no proven intervention exists, the use of placebo, or no intervention, is acceptable, or where for compelling and scientifically sound methodological reasons the use of any intervention less effective than the best proven one, the use of placebo or no intervention is necessary to determine the efficacy or safety of an intervention and the patients who receive any intervention less effective than the best proven one, placebo, or no intervention will not be subject to additional risks of serious or irreversible harm as a result of not receiving the best proven intervention.

Extreme care must be taken to avoid abuse of this option.

Post-trial provisions

34) In advance of a clinical trial, *sponsors, researchers and host country governments should make provisions for post-trial access for all participants* who still need an intervention identified as beneficial in the trial. This information must also be disclosed to participants during the informed consent process.

Research registration and publication and dissemination of results

35) Every research study involving human subjects must be registered in a publicly accessible database before recruitment of the first subject.

36) Researchers, authors, sponsors, editors and publishers all have ethical obligations with regard to the publication and dissemination of the results of research. *Researchers have a duty to make the results of their research on human subjects publicly available and are accountable for the completeness and accuracy of their reports.* All parties should adhere to accepted guidelines for ethical reporting. Negative and inconclusive as well as positive results must be published or otherwise made publicly available. Sources of funding, institutional affiliations and conflicts of interest must be declared in the publication. *Reports of research not in accordance with the principles of this Declaration should not be accepted for publication.*

Unproven interventions in clinical practice

37) In the treatment of an individual patient, where proven interventions do not exist or other known interventions have been ineffective, the physician, after seeking expert advice, with informed consent from the patient or a legally authorized representative, may use an unproven intervention if in the physician's judgment it offers hope of saving life, re-establishing health or alleviating suffering. This intervention should subsequently be made the object of research, designed to evaluate its safety and efficacy. In all cases, new information must be recorded and, where appropriate, made publicly available.

6.4. Ethics for engineers

There is no single ethics rule for the engineering community, but this issue is evolving rapidly. Even if the subject has already been broached, the issues raised by artificial intelligence make it a hot topic for the community. A complete description of the subject would be beyond the scope of this book, but it is useful to build some bridges between the medical world and the engineering one.

In Canada, convinced that young graduating engineers needed a standard of ethics and a ritual, Professor H.E.T. Haultain, University of Toronto, asked R. Kipling to write the Ritual of the Calling of an Engineer in 1922. The rituals are nowadays maintained by the Corporation of the Seven Wardens (https://ironring.ca/). It includes Kipling's oath, named the "Obligation of an Engineer":

> I am an Engineer. In my profession, I take deep pride. To it, I owe solemn obligations. As an engineer, I pledge to practice integrity and fair dealing, tolerance and respect, and to uphold devotion to the standards and dignity of my profession. I will always be conscious that my skill carries with it the obligation to serve humanity by making the best use of the Earth's precious wealth. As an engineer, I shall participate in none but honest enterprises. When needed, my skill and knowledge shall be given, without reservation, for the public good. In the performance of duty, and in fidelity to my profession, I shall give my utmost.

Another important reference should be the Archimedes Oath, proposed by the Ecole Polytechnique Fédérale de Lausanne (Switzerland):

– considering the life of Archimedes of Syracuse, who has illustrated the ambiguous potential of technology since Antiquity;

– considering the growing responsibility of engineers and scientists toward societies and nature;

– considering the importance of the ethical problems stemming from technology and its applications.

Today, I commit to the following statements and shall endeavor to reach toward the ideal that they represent:

– I shall practice for the good of humankind, respecting human rights[8] and the environment.

– I shall recognize the responsibility for my actions, after informing myself to the best of my abilities, and shall in no case discharge my responsibilities on another person.

– I shall endeavor to perfect my professional abilities.

– When choosing and implementing projects, I shall remain wary of their context and their consequences, notably in their technical, economic, social and ecological aspects. I shall give particular attention to projects with military applications.

– I shall contribute, to the extent of my abilities, to promote equitable relationships between people and to support the development of economically weaker countries.

– I shall transmit, with rigor and honesty, to discerningly chosen interlocutors, any important

8 According to the Universal Declaration of Human Rights of the United Nations (December 10, 1948).

information, if it constitutes a gain for society or if its retention constitutes a danger for others. In the latter case, I shall ensure that the communication yields concrete action.

– I shall not let myself be governed by the defense of my own interests or those of my corporation.

– I shall endeavor, to the best of my abilities, to lead my company to take into account the preoccupations of the present oath.

– I shall practice my profession in complete intellectual honesty, with conscience and dignity.

– I solemnly take this oath, freely and on my honor.

In both cases, the personal responsibility toward humanity and the scientific integrity strongly fit into the medical field. Following these ethics rules, engineers must consider the medical recommendation and follow it.

QUIZ.–

1) *Medical ethics rules were defined in the Nuremberg Code. Any clinical trial designer should exclusively refer to it.*

☐ Yes ☐ No

2) *A company wants to bring to the market a new device with (possible) increased performances compared to an existing solution. A clinical trial is envisaged against placebo. Is this solution convenient referring to ethics rules?*

☐ Yes ☐ No

3) *If no further use is expected (scientific publication, notified body files), is it possible to perform a clinical study without ethics committee approval?*

□ Yes □ No

4) *A clinical trial on a new artificial heart is carried out at a university hospital. A patient is admitted to hospital after a heart attack. The heart has been damaged dramatically and the patient's life is at stake. The surgeon wants to implant the artificial heart under study, but cannot obtain written consent. Should they proceed with the artificial heart operation anyway?*

□ Yes □ No

7

Clinical Trials Process

7.1. Clinical trials in the design process

7.1.1. *Before clinical testing*

When seeking the best efficiency and security for a medical device, results on humans are obviously the last level of proof that could be brought. These results derive from a long development process that starts with the ideation and first prototypes, but also overall numerical modeling, physical testing to verify the envisaged solution, sometimes in vitro testing and/or animal testing for the first validation purpose.

This chapter is dedicated to clinical trails on humans, but some key data on animal testing are given here. It should be pointed out that scientists face the same kind of ethics issues with animal testing, with a constant social questioning of the relevance of such trials. Basically, W. M. S. Russell and R. L. Burch established the three Rs (3Rs) as guiding principles for improved ethics in the use of animals in 1959:

– replace the use of animals in research whenever it is possible;

– reduce the number of animals by using more powerful methods or getting more information from the same cohort of animals;

– refinement: alleviate or minimize potential pain, suffering or distress, and enhance animal welfare for the animals.

The Council of Europe adopted the Treaty No. 123 "*European Convention for the Protection of Vertebrate Animals used for Experimental and other Scientific Purposes*" in 1986[1], which was converted into the *EU Directive 2010/63/EU (Sept. 22nd 2010) on the protection of animals used for scientific purposes* (EUR-Lex 2010). The EU Directive recognizes the necessity of animal testing, while strictly limiting the field of application (including applied research for medical purpose) and promoting alternative approaches.

The EU directive leaves the way open to a higher national ethics regulation. As an example, in France, a research project using animals is submitted to an authorization, after being evaluated by an Animal Ethics Committee. Any organization using animals for scientific purposes must be accredited, and people must have the necessary training. The choice of the animal species must be justified, and the animal origin identified. Then, researchers will have to follow the 3Rs principles in particular in reducing the number of animals and the suffering and distress.

Finally, researchers and engineers can also refer to the ISO 10993-2:2022 "*Biological evaluation of medical devices – Part 2: Animal welfare requirements*".

1 Available at: https://www.coe.int/en/web/conventions/full-list?module=treaty-detail&treatynum=123.

7.1.2. *Institutional guidelines*

Clinical testing is a key element in the design of medical devices. If it is well designed and conducted, the clinical testing gives a clinical proof of safety and efficiency of the device and helps to make the conditions of use (posology) as well as the limitations (adverse effects) more precise. In some cases, in spite of the efforts in pre-clinical testing or scientific proof approach, a device project could be discarded.

Moreover, the clinical proof (in pre-clinics, in clinics) is a major concern for the regulatory agencies to accept a medical device. The European Union has published three guides helping in clinical methodology[2]:

– MEDDEV 2.7/1 clinical evaluation: a guide for manufacturers and notified bodies;

– MEDDEV 2.7/4 guidelines on clinical investigations: a guide for manufacturers and notified bodies;

– MEDDEV 2.12/2 post market clinical follow-up studies.

In the United States, the FDA's main sources for medical devices clinical studies are as follows[3]:

– information sheet guidance for IRBs, clinical investigators, and sponsors: frequently asked questions about medical devices;

– information sheet guidance for IRBs, clinical investigators, and sponsors: significant risk and nonsignificant risk medical device studies.

2 For EU guidelines, see: https://ec.europa.eu/growth/sectors/medical-devices/current-directives/guidance_en.

3 For FDA guidance, see: https://www.fda.gov/regulatory-information/search-fda-guidance-documents/frequently-asked-questions-about-medical-devices, https://www.fda.gov/regulatory-information/search-fda-guidance-documents/significant-risk-and-nonsignificant-risk-medical-device-studies.

Lastly, the designers can refer to the international standards, such as the ISO 14155:2020 "Clinical investigation of medical devices for human subjects – Good clinical practice"[4]. This is the ISO implementation of ethics international rules as stated in the Declaration of Helsinki (see section 6.3) standing clearly for the responsibilities of the sponsor and the principal investigator, and putting the clinical trials in the background of risk evaluation.

7.1.3. *Clinical trials before going to market (EU – MEDDEV 2.7/1)*

Clinical testing is used before the device goes to market, and after, throughout its lifetime. Before authorization to go to market, clinical evaluation is used to demonstrate the safety and performance of each indication the supplier claims for the medical device. Clinical evaluation consists of a critical analysis of relevant clinical data that follow quality rules (well-funded methodology, good practices in statistics and respect of ethics rules).

In practice, clinical testing can refer to tests specifically designed for the medical device, published clinical testing on equivalent devices or other internal sources referring to clinical studies on equivalent devices, even unpublished. Whatever the situation, the sponsor of a clinical trial (a university hospital, the company that proposes a medical device) is responsible for the relevance of clinical data.

Clinical data obtained before going to market ought to be used in the leaflet of the new device for the indications claimed by supplier, contraindications, safety precautions and adverse reactions.

4 Available at: https://www.iso.org/standard/71690.html.

The EU document "MEDDEV 2.7.1" gives an example of a clinical evaluation report for the pre-market (clinical proof) and post-market (clinical follow-up). Even if the EU expects a clinical evaluation for each medical device, whatever the category, if the clinical evaluation is not appropriate to demonstrate the core requirement, the absence of a clinical evaluation must be thoroughly justified (ANSM 2017; EUR-Lex 2017).

7.1.4. *Bibliographically-based clinical proof and demonstration of equivalence*

A clinical trial based on previously published works is a relevant scientific review analyzing technical characteristics, objective, security and performance regarding the medical device. In this case, the demonstration is mainly based on clinical results obtained on an equivalent device, but can also include original results for the medical device.

A device can be considered as equivalent to another device if it is (MEDDEV 2.7/1, Chapter 5.1 (b)):

– clinically equivalent (indication, site of use, targeted population, clinical performances, etc.);

– technically equivalent (design, specification, operating mode, etc.);

– biologically equivalent (biocompatibility, tissues, materials, etc.).

The demonstration of equivalence is tedious work that should describe every point listed above, even the different versions of the equivalent device; therefore, the strict equivalence between two devices is very uncommon. In case of differences, the new medical device developer must justify that these differences have no impact on the performances and safety. Once demonstrated, the developer can use the clinical results from the equivalent medical device for their own proposed device. The equivalence can be sought at the early design stages, when performing the market analysis or prior to the art search.

Additionally, EU rules reinforce the role of clinical trials for class III and implantable devices; specific clinical trials are mandatory, even if equivalence can be demonstrated and used for some specific aspects of the demonstration.

7.1.5. *Clinical trials after going to market (EU – MDR2017 and EU – MEDDEV 2.12-1 rev 8)*

Post-market surveillance (PMS) must be contemplated and described in the pre-market files. The manufacturer must systematically survey the medical device data obtained since they have been produced. A voluntary and organized information system should collect clinical data usable for reinforcing security and performance of the medical device.

The EU expects the manufacturer to regularly update the clinical evaluation after going to market and all along the medical device lifetime; documentation must be updated as well. New data for updating can come from equivalent devices as well as from the given device. They consist of a literature review and clinical studies (clinical investigations, observational clinical studies, registries, etc.). Obviously, a clinical study that starts before market approval can be pursued after it has been approved, especially to look for long-term effects. This aspect is common for implantable devices.

Moreover, the post-market clinical follow-up (PMCF) should clarify risk levels, help in identifying or discarding hazards and therefore modify the risk analysis. The PMCF ought to be designed before market approval with specialists in statistics and clinics.

7.2. Insight: MDR2017 and the French implementation

In the European Community, the mandatory regulatory framework for medical devices is the EU-MDR2017. As a regulation of the EU Parliament and the Council, it prevails on national laws.

Then, within EU-MDR2017, clinical investigation differs depending on the risk for the patient/subjects, evaluated from the class of medical device and the presence of a CE mark. If the risk is considered high enough for the patient, a scientific evaluation (Agence nationale de sécurité du médicament et des produits de santé (ANSM)) is mandatory, otherwise an ethics evaluation by an institutional review board (IRB) (Comité de Protection de la Personne) is supposed to be sufficient.

The risk level for most of the systems is described in the EU-MDR2017. The key elements are shown in Figure 7.1. The risk associated with a medical device depends on the type of device: invasive, non-invasive, implantable or active; the type of interaction of the device with the body: biological, chemical, absorbable, ionizing, energy transfer; the targeted system, with higher risk for the circulatory system and the nervous system; the duration of use, with higher risk for long-term use.

Another important issue is the objective of the clinical investigation. Is the objective to obtain the medical device conformity? Then, the clinical investigation purpose should be to establish or verify (i) that the device reaches the intended performances in normal conditions, (ii) the clinical benefits for the patient and (iii) the clinical safety and identification of side effects in normal use. Clinical trials out of these objectives are still possible under each country's management. In France, the ANSM has not published updated conditions. All classification rules are shown in Figure 7.2.

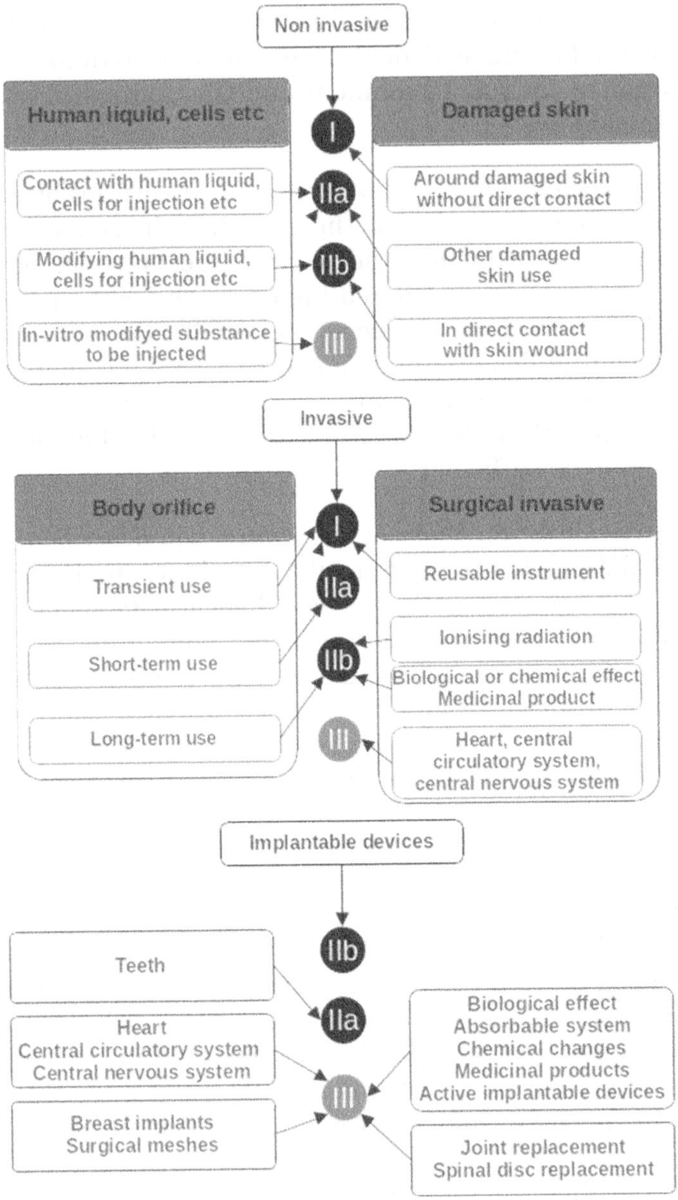

Non invasive
Human liquid, cells etc
Contact with human liquid, cells for injection etc
Modifying human liquid, cells for injection etc
In-vitro modifyed substance to be injected
I
IIa
IIb
III
Damaged skin
Around damaged skin without direct contact
Other damaged skin use
In direct contact with skin wound
Invasive
Body orifice
Transient use
Short-term use
Long-term use
I
IIa
IIb
III
Surgical invasive
Reusable instrument
Ionising radiation
Biological or chemical effect Medicinal product
Heart, central circulatory system, central nervous system
Implantable devices
IIb
IIa
III
Teeth
Heart
Central circulatory system
Central nervous system
Breast implants
Surgical meshes
Biological effect
Absorbable system
Chemical changes
Medicinal products
Active implantable devices
Joint replacement
Spinal disc replacement

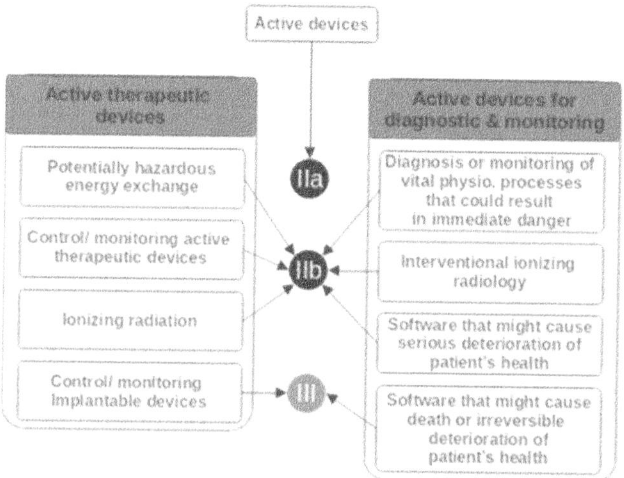

Figure 7.1. *Risk classification in EU-MDR2017. For a color version of this figure, see www.iste.co.uk/molimard/biomedicaldevices.zip*

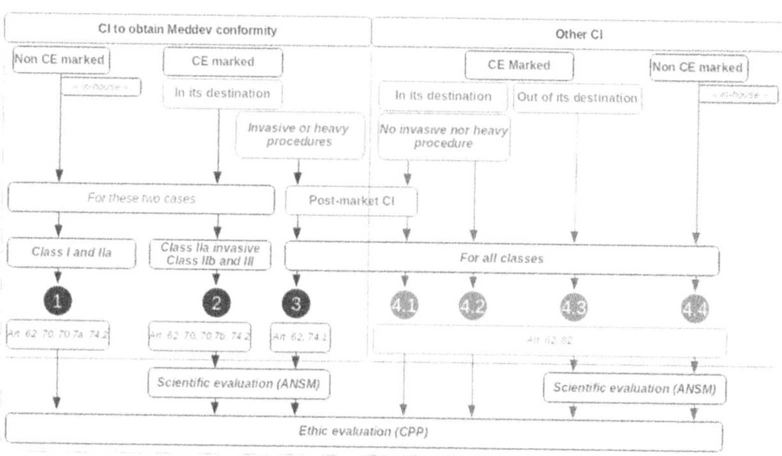

Figure 7.2. *Clinical investigation classification in France after EU-MDR2017. For a color version of this figure, see www.iste.co.uk/molimard/biomedicaldevices.zip*

For all clinical investigation, data are collected, then a CNIL[5] authorization (or MR001 formula) is mandatory. All other rules deriving from ethics are not detailed here, but must be fulfilled (e.g. patient written consent and vigilance). Lastly, the promoter must take out insurance.

Besides the EU rules, in France, the ethics rules are regulated by the Loi Jardé (Jardé's law). The EU-MDR2017 rules prevail for medical devices. Out of the medical devices context, the Loi Jardé is valid for all clinical trials that are not related to medical devices, as defined by EU-MDR2017.

We can assess that if the object under study is a specific response of the human body, and if a medical device is used as a means for this study, then the Loi Jardé is the right regulatory framework. However, if the object under study is the medical device itself, then EU-MDR2017 must be used.

Following the Loi Jardé, clinical trials are divided into investigations involving human persons (Recherches impliquant la personne humaine (RIPH)) and other investigations.

Other investigations could be, for example, a processing database with personal information or cosmetics, sports or a social science survey. The main point in any case is personal data protection, and the Reference Methodology MR003 must be respected (CNIL MR003). Moreover, in the case of a multicentric retrospective clinical study, a research authorization from CEREES (Expert Committee for Health Research, Studies and Evaluations) must be obtained beforehand. If possible, written information is given to the patient/subject and they have to give their consent in some specific cases (recording on ethnic group, religion, genetics, political opinion, morals). The principal investigator is not

5 The CNIL (National Commission on Informatics and Liberty) is an independent French administrative regulatory body whose mission is to ensure that data privacy law is applied.

necessarily a physician. Lastly, any biological collection collected during the study must be declared to the Ministry of Research.

RIPH investigations differ, depending on the risk for the patient/subjects. The lowest risk level, RIPH3, is "non-interventional prospective studies". This means that the study does not change the clinical protocol. If something in the protocol has to be changed, for example, extra measurement, or the specific use of a medical device (e.g. an orthesis), then it goes to "interventional studies" (RIPH1) or to "minimal risks and stresses" (RIPH2). The difference between these last two lies in the risk for the patient. RIPH1 and RIPH2 need explicit consent from the patient/subject in almost every case. Then, the reference methodology used is CNIL MR001. Written information has to be provided to the patient/subject. For RIPH1 levels, the principal investigator is necessarily a clinician (physician, dentist or midwife); the list opens up to other "qualified persons" for RIPH2 and RIPH3. Insurance is mandatory (RIPH1 and RIPH2). In the case of RIPH3, the risk being lower, the procedure only involves written information, without explicit consent (except for data collection of ethnic group, religion, genetics, political opinion and morals), and insurance is not mandatory.

The realization of clinical trials must be done under a certified environment, as stated in Article L. 1121-13 of the Public Health Code[6]:

> Research can only be carried out in a facility that has human, material and technical resources adapted to the research and compatible with the safety of the persons involved.

6 Available at: http://www.legifrance.gouv.fr/affichCodeArticle.do?idArticle=LEGIARTI000036515061&cidTexte=LEGITEXT000006072665&dateTexte=20180119.

> This location must be authorized for a specific period of time, in the case of research mentioned in 1° of article L. 1121-1[7] outside places of care, as well as in hospital departments and in any other place where healthcare professionals practice when such research requires acts other than those they usually perform in the course of their work, or when such research is carried out on persons presenting a clinical condition distinct from that for which the department is responsible. This authorization is granted by the Director General of the regional health or by the Minister of Defense, if the site falls under his or her authority.

7.3. Classification of clinical trials

Clinical research can be classified according to the subject under study: treatment, diagnostic, prevention, quality of life, genetics, epidemiology or screening research. Medical device studies usually lie in the first two studies.

Another classification, specific to evaluating medication and devices, is related to the study objectives. They are *interventional studies*, as they consist of acting directly on a cohort, in contrast to *observational studies*, which use medical databases as inputs.

Clinical trials are commonly classified into four consecutive phases, addressing different concerns:

– Phase I trials: *is the treatment safe?* The goal is to evaluate the safety of the treatment, determine a safe dosage range and identify side effects. This first trial is conducted on small cohorts.

7 Investigations involving human persons (RIPH).

– Phase II trials: *is the treatment effective?* As the treatment is supposed to be safe, the group can be larger without major impact on security. Of course, in addition to efficacy, the safety is still being studied.

– Phase III trials: *is the treatment safe, effective and competitive?* As the first results on safety and effectiveness are convincing, a third study on large groups is carried out to confirm the effectiveness, monitor side effects, compare to gold standard treatments and collect information that will allow the experimental treatment to be used safely.

– Phase IV trials: *what happens in real life?* After the medical device is approved and proposed on the market, post-marketing studies are mandatory. They provide additional information on the risks, benefits and best use of the treatment.

Before starting a phase I clinical trial, numerical simulations, studies on bio-engineered tissues or animal testing are recommended. However, first steps on humans are difficult in the absence of previous works that could help in designing a clinical trial. Then, in addition to the classification of the clinical trials given above, a *feasibility study* might be necessary. This is composed of a set of small-scale explorations of the area of the proposed clinical trial (*pilot studies*). Each pilot study's main characteristics are that of an experimental clinical trial; it should evaluate the protocol, improve the study design and its primary outcome should be a cohort sample size.

The design of clinical trials is closely related to statistics and seeks to remove unexpected effects. Firstly, the question of objectivity of the patient, caregiver or statistician is addressed using *blind*, *double-blind* or *triple-blind* trials. By not revealing to participants the nature of what they are receiving, administering or observing, observation (expectancy) bias can be removed. This method is not adapted to *longitudinal studies*. In such a case, the patient is followed over time and repeated observations of the same variables are made. It is therefore ethically and practically impossible to blind the intervention. Such a trial is called an "*open-label clinical trial*".

A clinical trial can be performed per se, without comparison to a reference. This is called an *uncontrolled trial*, and all participants are in the same arm. However, it will attribute to the intervention every event occurring during the protocol, and in particular spontaneous recovery. For that reason, *controlled clinical trials* use a second arm as a control. The nature of this arm may vary depending on the study. "No treatment" might be an option, but in this case, it is impossible to perform a blind test. Then, a popular choice is the use of a placebo, which is an inactive intervention that mimics the intervention under study. In this case, blind tests are possible, but patients in the placebo arm do not receive treatments; that is ethically problematic. One way to limit this effect is to remove these patients from the study as soon as possible, but this limits the interpretation of results to a short time period. Finally, the ethically recommended situation consists of comparing the new treatment to the gold standard. Comparison to historical data, or dose comparison are also possible; usually, they are coupled to another controlled arm and constitute a third arm. Lastly, the *cross over design* consists of sequentially using the same participants in both situations. In this case, each participant is their own control, which is statistically interesting, as it reduces the inter subject bias. However, a cross over design is limited to stable diseases (e.g. chronic), with rapid effects for treatment as well as rapid reversibility after its interruption. A wash out period before the test begins and between the two situations should be considered. A variant of the cross over design is the *split body trial*. The controlled and the treatment situations are not studied sequentially, but they are applied on two similar organs, typically the left and right leg, or arm. This type of trial is commonly used in dermatology and ophthalmology.

Any clinical trial must be *randomized* to eliminate confounding factors. Randomization is the process of randomly assigning participants to either the treatment or the control arm. In the case of cross over design, the order of operations is defined randomly. Many strategies can be derived from randomization. In a *stratified randomization* scheme, randomization is applied to each stratum that corresponds to a prognostic variable. This method balances patient groups according to characteristics (covariate) considered to be a prognostic variable. In the same idea, *cluster randomization* considers each investigation site[8] (hospital, interventional group). Each site is considered as a unit of trial; randomization is balanced at the site level, and exploitation of the results is also possible at this level. *Block randomization* arranges experimental units into groups with similar properties, for example, same sex; in doing so, this property is controlled and the overall variability is reduced. As they add statistical degrees of freedom, the number of blocks, clusters, or strata must be limited.

As it can be observed, the trials can be carried out in *parallel groups*, meaning that each arm runs parallel to the other with no changes for a patient, or in *cross over*, each patient being successively in the controlled arm and the treatment arm. In the case of multiple interventions, methods derived from the design of experiments can be used, as *factorial design*. Results are analyzed with repeated measures analysis of variance (rANOVA).

Experimental studies can have different levels of scientific explanation. *Pragmatic clinical trials* focus on the correlation between treatments and outcomes, without looking for causality. They can be compared to *explanatory clinical trials*, which optimize the experimental conditions to study

8 A clinical trial is *unicentric* if it is performed in a single center, or *multicentric* if various centers are involved. Phases I and II are usually unicentric trials, but phase III is always multicentric.

whether and how an intervention works. The entire experiment must be designed to control for all known biases and confounders so that the effect of the intervention is maximized.

Clinical trials can be distinguished as a *prospective* or *retrospective* study. In the first case, results are recorded along time, with conditions that are optimized for the study. In the second one, results already exist, and they are post-processed in order to extract a result; in this case, conditions cannot be optimized. Experimental designs as described before are all prospective studies and they usually lie in phase I, II or III trials.

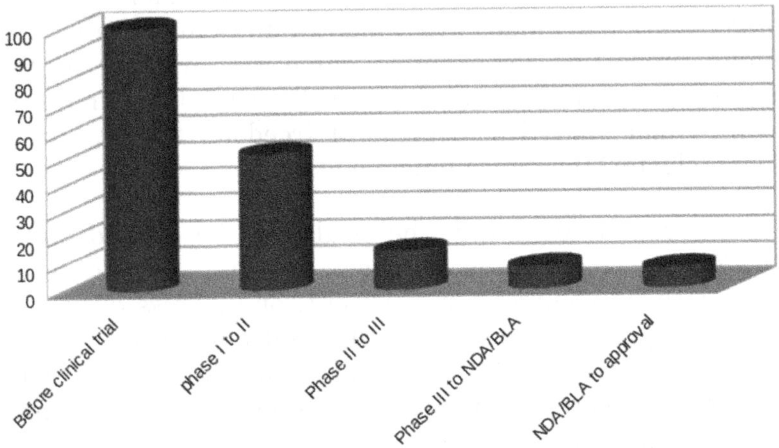

Figure 7.3. *Cumulative success rate for drugs during clinical trial phases (Thomas et al. 2021). For a color version of this figure, see www.iste.co.uk/molimard/biomedicaldevices.zip*

Lastly, it is almost impossible to collect clear data with medical devices, but the clinical development success rate for drugs shows that only 7% of drugs starting with clinical trials are finally approved. Even though these data strongly depend on the medical field, the crucial step is the first one (safety level, see below).

7.4. Insight: the ISO 14155

Compared to ICH-GCP, the ISO 14155 good clinical practices are both a highly ethical standard by including ethical considerations from the Declaration of Helsinki in its current implementation and a quality insurance process. The ISO 14155 gives more practical rules than the Nuremberg Code or the Declaration of Helsinki, and describes the role of each stakeholder (subject, principal investigator, promoter, IRB, regulation body). Convergence with EU and U.S. regulations is assured.

7.4.1. *Ethics consideration*

The investigators must have a fluid communication with IRB. The IRB is also known as an independent ethics committee (IEC), but other denominations exist. In France, the Local Ethics Committee and the Personal Protection Committee are two forms of these IRB working at two levels (see section 7.2). Investigators must present an initial submission to the IRB, wait for a positive answer before starting the clinical investigation, communicate to the IRB any changes or events during the investigation, send intermediate reports and finally close the investigation with a final report. In case of changes or incidents, an explicit answer from the IRB should be necessary.

The initial submission must contain many planning documents: the clinical investigation plan; the investigator's brochure; the document provided to subjects, including the informed consent form; subject recruitment procedures; the curriculum vitae of the principal investigator. Depending on the design of the clinical investigation and national or regional requirements, other documents might be provided: the draft of the observation book; documents related to payments and compensation to subjects; the remuneration proposed to the institution or principal investigator;

documents relating to a possible conflict of interest; and a proof of assurance of clinical investigation.

Communication to the subjects is specifically addressed in the standard. Informed consent is obtained using an information form and a consent form.

The information form should explicitly state that the protocol is under research and give all necessary information on it (objective, duration, description of the medical device, procedures, investigation methodology) and on the benefits (for the patient and for the community) and risks (residual risks). It should indicate the medical alternative, the compensation to the subject (fee, supplementary treatments in case of complication), the role of each actor, conditions to stop and a contact person.

Each consent form must be obtained and stored before going to investigation, except in case of an emergency for the patient. The consent must be based on clear and complete information, given in an understandable language, and without any kind of undue incentive or excessive influence. The consent itself should explicitly state that a refusal would not cause any prejudice. It contains a consent for the use of personal data as well. In the case of a vulnerable subject (minor child, learning difficulties, etc.), the legal representative is in charge of giving their consent. The subject should have information according to their capacity to understand. For illiterate people, the consent can be obtained orally, after reading the information form, in the presence of a third party. Lastly, in case of emergency for the patient's life, and if the consent of a legal representative is impossible, the medical staff can decide on going to an experimental protocol, if the reference treatment advantages are not sufficient and if the use of the medical device under investigation is likely to eliminate the risk to the patient's life. In this case, the patient or their legal representative must be informed as soon as possible and the consent obtained before going further.

As it can be observed, the ISO14155 develops a quality insurance protocol that covers the ethics considerations.

7.4.2. *Planning of the clinical investigation*

Planning the clinical investigation consists of (1) knowing exactly the reason why this experiment is necessary, (2) developing a strategy that can statistically prove an effect and (3) communicating with authorities in the respect of the scientific good practices[9] and the patients. The global idea is that no one can expose people to a certain degree of risk without strong arguments on the probability of success.

The answer to the first concern is based on the state of the art, with the corresponding scientific literature and the technological background (patent, internal reports). Of course, the previous works done by the research team on the subject are of major interest. This could be computer modeling, cell engineering and pre-clinical trials on cadavers or animals. The state of the art helps in designing the clinical investigation; it should make researchers define the target population, identify possible confounding factors and design the best interventional test with its instrumentation.

The promoter of the research must provide various documents:

– The clinical investigation plan gives a detailed argumentation and description of the clinical investigation. It includes, in particular, the investigation place and justifies the choice for the patient safety and some practical

---

9 See: Global Hamonization Taskforce, Clinical Evaluation, SG5/N2R8:2007, http://www.imdrf.org/docs/ghtf/final/sg5/technical-docs/ghtf-sg5-n3-clinical-investigations-100212.pdf.

considerations (trained professionals on site, patients reachability).

– The booklet for the investigator summarizes relevant information to conduct the clinical trials and to orient the work in case of necessity. The booklet also details the role of a principal investigator.

– The observation notebook is a record of all information throughout the clinical investigation.

– A supervising plan for the follow-up of the clinical investigation is proposed in order to take a decision in case of problems during the study, such as serious adverse events (AEs). A supervising committee, composed of external scientific personalities, can inform the promoter.

The medical devices being prototypes, they must be clearly identified during the clinical investigation and exceeding material should be discarded.

7.4.3. *Clinical investigation follow-up*

A clinical investigation must not begin before completing the IRB authorization. It begins with a kick-off visit on each investigation site. Each investigator has to form a register describing their functions and the authorizations they will get for the investigation, and the place for the trials. The supervision of the clinical investigation begins as described in the supervising plan.

If any change occurs with respect to the produced documents, in particular, the experimental plan or the investigator booklet, amendments can be proposed to the principal investigator, to the promoter and to the IRB or regulation authorities for document under their approval. Accepted changes must be clearly recorded, with the date of the new version.

More generally, every document of the clinical investigation must be carefully stored and identified. Any change should be clearly readable (the new version as well as the old one). Due to confidentiality issues, the project stakeholders should only have access to necessary data for their task. A secured data management system should fulfill several requirements on security (e.g. access, antivirus software), integrity of the data, etc.

Every AE or medical device failure has to be carefully noted. AEs can be any unfavorable sign associated with the use of a medical investigational product, whether related to the medical investigational product or not. AEs are classified as an AE or a serious adverse event (SAE), depending on the severity. An SAE is defined as an event related to a clinical trial that can result (1) in death, (2) is life threatening, (3) requires patient hospitalization or causes prolongation of existing hospitalization, (4) results in persistent or significant disability/incapacity, (5) may have caused a congenital anomaly/birth defect, (6) requires intervention to prevent permanent impairment or damage, or (7) any other serious important medical events[10]. If the event is related to the device itself, the (S)AE becomes a (serious) adverse device effect ((S)ADE) and if the event could not be suspected before experiments, the event is "unexpected" and the SADE can therefore be considered an unexpected serious adverse device effect.

In the same philosophy, any medical device defect must be notified, even if no adverse event occurred. The defect can be related to the reliability, the security, performance or even identification. The failure analysis should discuss the possibility of an adverse event.

10 From the FDA: https://www.fda.gov/safety/reporting-serious-problems-fda/what-serious-adverse-event.

A register of subjects must be maintained. In the spirit of confidentiality, it contains the identification keys for each patient. Personal data must be stored in a secured manner, and only authorized people should have access to it. They must be respected in reports and publications. If a subject leaves the study, the reason must be written in the observation notebook.

7.4.4. *Ending a clinical investigation*

The interruption or the end of a clinical investigation can occur prematurely in an individual site, or in all the clinical sites, if an unacceptable risk is suspected. The initiative may come from the promoter, the principal investigator, the IRB or a regulatory body. The stakeholders must communicate their decision to the others, including the subjects. Even in the case of interruption or premature end, the promoter is still responsible for the means associated with the clinical investigation. In case of interruption, the clinical investigation can resume if the corrective actions are made, explained to the IRB and regulatory body, and after acceptance by these two.

A routine closing is done when all the investigation documents are completed and stored, the exceeding medical devices are discarded and all the stakeholders are notified.

The principal investigator must write a clinical investigation report and transmit this to the promoter, the IRB and the regulation body. It is a scientific report, recalling the methodology, the clinical investigation design, the results (respecting the subjects privacy), the statistical analysis and a critical appreciation of the results with respect to the objectives of the investigation. The report must also contain the deviations from the clinical investigation plan and the list of medical devices used. The promoter and the principal investigator should keep records of the whole investigation.

It is highly recommended to publish the results, even if they are negative. This can be in regular scientific journals and/or in a dedicated database, such as clinicaltrials.gov.

QUIZ.– A company wants to develop a smart watch to monitor blood pressure, blood saturation and heart rate. They want to qualify the device as CE medical.

1) *What classification would you propose?*

□ Class I □ Class IIa

□ Class IIb □ Class III

2) *In the context of the EU, will they need a notified body approval?*

□ Yes □ No

3) *In the context of the EU, is it necessary to go for a clinical trial?*

□ Yes □ No □ Depends

4) *After a rigorous bibliographical analysis, the developers did not find any instrument comparable enough for a demonstration of equivalence. They decided to go for a first clinical trial. What would be the most appropriate denomination?*

□ Feasibility study □ Phase I □ Phase II

□ Phase III □ Phase IV

5) *During the test, a group of volunteers will wear the device (and the results will be recorded) during a whole day; at the beginning and at the end of the day, results will be compared with a ground truth value given by a reference protocol (blood test).*

How would you qualify the test?

☐ Randomized ☐ Blind

☐ Parallel groups ☐ Cross over

6) *How consent will be obtained?*

☐ As we asked for volunteers, no more consent is necessary

☐ Written consent ☐ Oral consent

7) *The researcher defends the project, mentioning that the main advantage of this trial is advances in science and technology. Would this argument be enough to convince the IRB to authorize the clinical trial?*

☐ Yes ☐ No

8

Introduction to Biostatistics

8.1. Introduction

Because of the high variability between humans, a treatment (drug, medical device, etc.) must show its efficiency and safety on a cohort of patients in a clinical trial. The efficiency will then only have a statistical meaning. Biostatistics is a complete approach that helps in designing a clinical trial to get meaningful results, that is, a statistically significant difference (if any) while removing statistical bias. A huge amount of literature can be read about biostatistics, showing the importance and also the level of complexity behind it. Here, only a few aspects representative of the most common situations will be mentioned.

8.2. Selection rules for statistical processing

Dealing with random variables will be tricky if the experiment is badly designed, that is, if the question to answer is not explicitly posed, and confounding factors are not clarified. The decision tree shown in Figure 8.1 gives the main orientation for this. We must answer the following questions:

– Are the data quantitative or qualitative?

– Do we want to see a difference between situations or a relationship between parameters?

– How many groups are there?

– How many independent variables or predictors are there?

– Are the samples dependent or independent?

– How much do we know about the distribution?

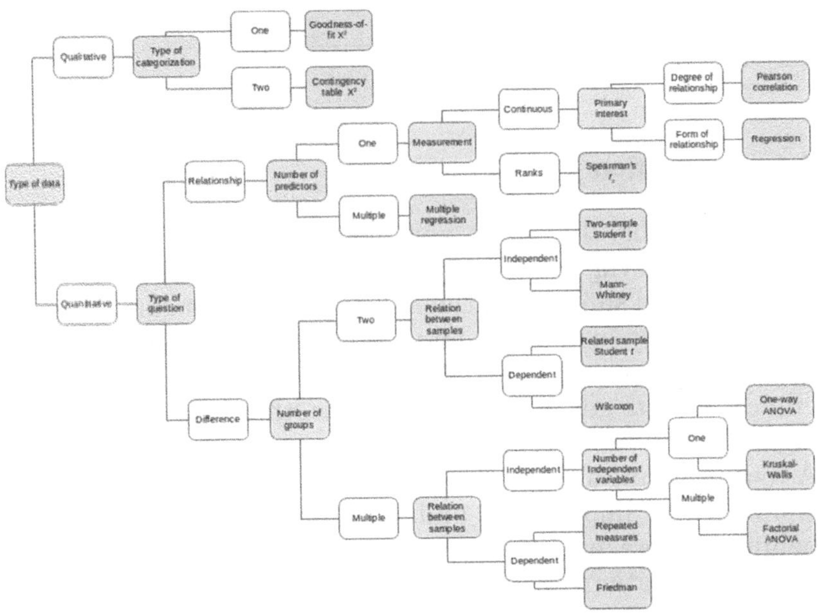

Figure 8.1. *Decision tree for statistical test. For a color version of this figure, see www.iste.co.uk/molimard/biomedicaldevices.zip*

As an output, the decision tree gives statistical tests (X^2, Pearson correlation, regression, Spearman test, Student's *t*-test, Mann–Whitney, Wilkoxon test, analysis of variance (ANOVA), Krustal–Wallis test and Freidman test). All of these tests are pre-implemented in general numerical computing software (Matlab/Octave or Python), statistics software (R, JASP) or even spreadsheets (Excel, LibreOffice Calc). The reader should refer to specialized books to explore all of these possibilities (and many more than these!). Here, we will focus on the most common situation, which is to compare two sets of data and determine if they are statistically equal, and regression analysis.

8.3. Hypothesis testing

8.3.1. *General principle on hypothesis testing*

How can we conclude that a medical treatment has a positive or negative effect? In practice, this very often means comparing the averages of two test groups for sets of results of generally different sizes and dispersion. Hypothesis testing makes it possible to answer this type of question in a context where a random variation of the studied property, due to measurement noise or batch variability for example, is not negligible compared to the desired variation.

To perform hypothesis testing, it is necessary to define an H_0 hypothesis and its H_1 alternative. Interestingly, the way to write the hypothesis is never “the effect of the proposed treatment is different from the reference treatment” as the sponsor of a study would say, but on the contrary the H_0 hypothesis should be “the effect of the proposed treatment and the reference one has no difference”. The reason for that is that it is possible to prove equality, but not a difference. Then the logic is to determine that it is impossible to prove an equality, and therefore, the difference is the most probable.

This assumption must be formalized as a mathematical test, usually written as:

$$T = \Delta E / \sigma(\Delta E) \qquad [8.1]$$

This test compares the difference of two means (ΔE) and the combined standard deviation of these means ($\sigma(\Delta E)$). In order to define a criterion for acceptance or rejection of the test, a probability level stating the risk of an error must be defined and thus the statistical distribution. Of course, the distribution is only known through realizations: they can be used to test the accordance to known statics (Gaussian distribution, log-normal distribution, etc.).

In any case, the methodology must be written beforehand, and the acceptance level is decided prior to clinical testing. Finally, after the tests are carried out, conclusions are drawn.

The designer of a clinical test should face two classical but important situations: the first one consists of comparing two statistically independent groups, for example, men and women. Then, the test will make the *difference of the two means* as described before. But the two groups can also be statistically dependent, typically with or without a medical device. In this case, the inter-patient variability can be greatly compensated considering for each patient the difference (with/without the medical device) and comparing the *mean difference* to zero. The first situation is known as an unpaired test and the second one as a paired test. By removing the inter-patient variability, the paired test is likely to be more sensitive than the unpaired test.

Lastly, problems can arise when a statistical dependence is not identified or not taken into account. In the paired situation introduced above (with/without a medical device), the way to conduct the experiment is crucial. If tests are performed systematically first with the medical device and second without, a temporal effect (the learning curve of the test for the patient) should bias the results. Therefore, in this case, it is recommended to randomize the order of the tests. This error is known as a *confounding factor*.

In the first case (man/woman), other errors may occur. If the mean age of the population of men and women is different, then the difference observed during the test should be related to the sex, but also to the age. This is *selection bias*. One possible way to treat this error is to adjust the means (and reject patients); another one consists of multivariate analysis, taking into account both factors. In every case, the test will lose sensitivity.

Other kinds of errors may occur during clinical trials: if some of the patients leave the protocol, this may impact the results, and even inverse the trends when considering only those who finish the protocol. In order to remove this error (*attrition bias*), the good treatment should be on the initial cohort. This is called an *in the intent-to-treat* analysis.

Maybe one of the most prevalent error sources is the researcher themselves. As they are personally and professionally involved in the work, they want to obtain a positive result and could orient – even unconsciously – the study: for example, in processing data before the end or by paying more attention to one group than the other. One way to discard this bias (*assessment bias*) is to work in a *blind experiment* (neither the patient nor the practitioner knows the group) and to have a statistical analysis performed by a third party outside the research group.

To reduce possible bias, this blinding principle is usually extended to the patient, and to the statistician in charge of analyzing the results, giving *double-blind* or *triple-blind* trials.

The result of the statistical test is "I can *certainly* reject the H_0 hypothesis". *Certain* here means in a statistical sense, that is, with a defined level of risk, generally 5%. Hypothesis tests are therefore to be used in an uncertain context, because of the dispersion of the measures or because of the limited information available. This type of test therefore makes it possible to discriminate between factors that may have an effect and factors that may not. However, there is no indication of the intensity of the effect, and we can conclude that a result for a given treatment is statistically different to another one, but maybe this should have no sufficient effect on the patient. It is only a question of balance between the mean and the standard deviation, and an interpretation of the result in a more physical/medical way is necessary.

8.3.2. *Error of the first and second king, power of a test*

As stated above, statistical certainty is a challenging concept. It is possible that the test gives a "rejection" result, which is false, for example, because the sample contains elements that are statistically sparse. This is the error of the first kind, also called the α error. Similarly, it is possible that the test gives a "no rejection" result when the hypothesis should be rejected. This alternative error is the error of the second kind, called the β error. Table 8.1 presents the different possible situations. Although more difficult to handle, the β error is of great practical importance. Indeed, the non-rejection of a hypothesis that should be rejected means that the test used is not discriminatory. Note that $(1 - \beta)$ is called the *power of the test* because it quantifies the test's ability to provide useful information (rejection).

A test becomes more powerful when the dispersion is reduced: increasing the power of the test therefore corresponds to the following.

– Work on measurement tools by reducing measurement error.

– Resume operating conditions in order to limit dispersion, for example, by eliminating inter-batch variability, better controlling environmental conditions (temperature and humidity) or reducing the cohort variability working on the exclusion criteria.

– Increase the number of tests so that the dispersion over the mean is reduced and the statistical law is better controlled. It should be noted, however, that the dispersion over the mean varies only in $1/\sqrt{N}$, which implies a lot of effort for a limited result.

H_0 hypothesis	Accept	Reject
True	Right decision (true positive)	False positive Error of the first kind (α)
False	False negative Error of the second kind (β)	Right decision (true negative)

Table 8.1. *Error of the first and second kind*

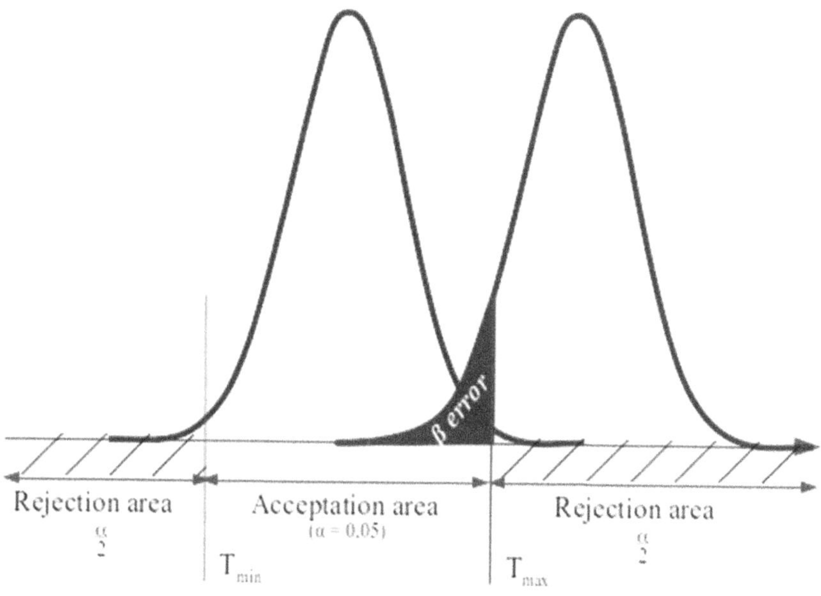

Figure 8.2. *Graphical representation of the error of the second kind. For a color version of this figure, see www.iste.co.uk/molimard/biomedicaldevices.zip*

Despite its practical importance, it is not possible to know by definition the true value of the *t*-test and it is strictly impossible to qualify β and (1 – β). An estimate is nevertheless possible, assuming a minimum desirable deviation between two sets of measurements. By giving the number of tests and a standard deviation for each case, it is quite possible to know the upper value T_{max} of the confidence interval associated with the H_0 hypothesis, and then the probability level associated with the true distribution, for the T_{max} value (Figure 8.2). Finally, since the essential parameter is the number of tests in each case, the minimum number of tests necessary to discriminate between the two averages can be established. This approach is a predictive approach, based on many hypotheses, but which has the advantage of discussing a priori the feasibility of a study. In the traditional way, the power of the test is adjusted to 80%.

NOTE 8.1.– The true positive rate is also called the sensitivity ($Sensitivity = \frac{\sum true\ positive}{\sum true\ positive + false\ negative}$) of the test and the false positive rate the fall-out ($fall - out = \frac{\sum false\ positive}{\sum false\ positive + false\ true\ negative}$) $= 1 - specificity$. The curve representing the sensitivity versus the fall-out is called the receiver operating characteristic (ROC) curve (Figure 8.3). The slope 1 line represents 50% error, and so a purely random behavior. Therefore, the further the ROC curve is to the slope 1 curve, the better the test selectivity.

NOTE 8.2.– Many considerations other than this technical aspect are included in the definition of the number of tests. For example, in clinical investigations, patient safety limits the number of trials. Indeed, the larger the number of patients, the greater the likelihood of having an adverse side effect.

NOTE 8.3.– Increasing the power of a test, to make the result statistically significant, allows smaller deviations to be discriminated. The physical meaning behind the experimental methodology must not be lost. This gap could be so small that its practical importance is null, even if it is statistically significant.

NOTE 8.4.– Increasing the number of experiments to get statistically significant results is considered as a scientific misconduct called “p-hacking”. This comes from a questionable practice in many papers that focus on results with statistically significant differences, leaving apart the others. Again, this is considered to be a scientific misconduct: from the good practice point of view, both positive and negative results should be commented in the same way.

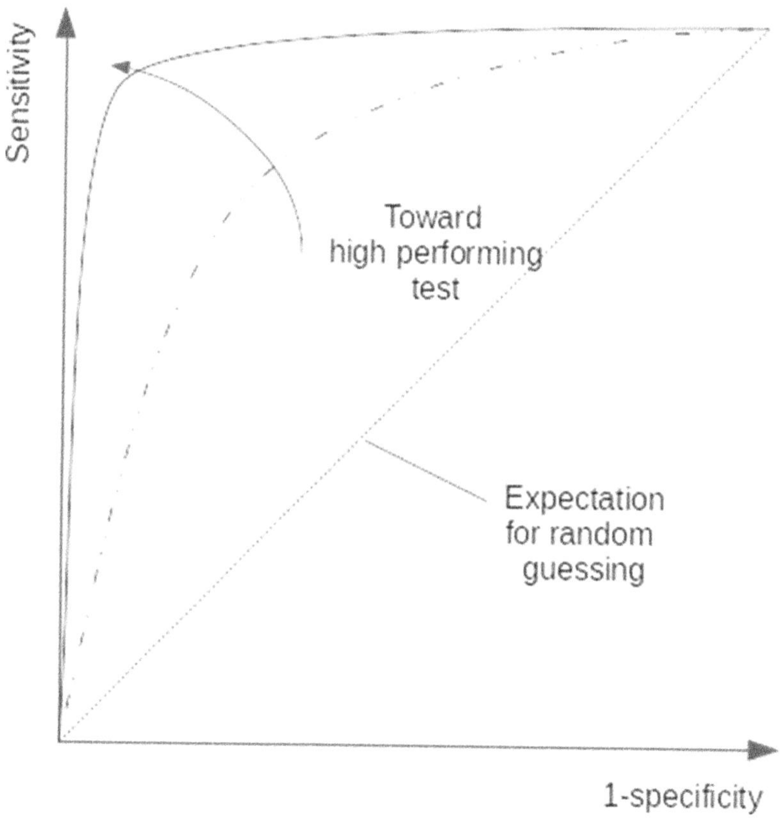

Figure 8.3. *ROC curve. For a color version of this figure, see www.iste.co.uk/molimard/biomedicaldevices.zip*

8.3.3. *Comparing two sets of variables: parametric or nonparametric testing*

The central limit theorem assumes that the statistical law followed by a sum of random events of any statistical law tends toward the normal law. This very important result is obviously applicable to the average. If the number of random events is not high enough, deviations from the normal distribution can become significant, which is the case in most experiments.

At this stage, two cases can be identified: in the first case, random events follow a normal law; then, for a limited numbers of points, Student's law and the Student's test (a.k.a. *t*-test) can be used. But if no argument can be made for a normal distribution, or if the distribution is clearly different, nonparametric tests should be used. Many tests exist, for example, the Mann–Whitney and Wilcoxon tests (a.k.a. *U*-test).

The following tests can assess the distribution normality: D'Agostino's K-squared test, Jarque–Bera test, Anderson–Darling test, Cramer–von Mises criterion, Kolmogorov–Smirnov test, Lilliefors test, Shapiro–Wilk test and Pearson's chi-squared test. In 2011, a study compared the Shapiro–Wilk, Kolmogorov–Smirnov, Lilliefors and Anderson–Darling tests and concluded that Shapiro–Wilk has the best power for a given significance (Razali and Wah 2011); others focused on the Jarque–Bera test (Thadewald and Büning 2007).

The Jarque–Bera test is the third and fourth standardized moments of the actual distribution to that of a normal distribution. The third standardized moments, the skewness $(\frac{1}{n}\sum(x_i - \bar{x})^3)/\sigma^3$ quantifies the symmetry of the distribution and the fourth standardized moment, the kurtosis $(\frac{1}{n}\sum(x_i - \bar{x})^4)/\sigma^4$, the distance of the realizations to the mean.

The Shapiro–Wilk test compares the distance to the mean value $\sum_{i=1}^{n}(x_i - \bar{x})^2$ to the weighted sum of the order statistics (i.e. the difference between the ith higher value and the ith lower value) $(\sum_{i=1}^{n}(a_i x_{(i)}))^2$. a_i weights contain information on normal distribution $(a_{1,} \ldots a_n) = \frac{m^T v^{-1}}{C}$, where m is the expected value of the order statistics of (independent and identically distributed) random variables sampled from the standard normal distribution, v is the covariance matrix of those normal order statistics and C is the vector norm of $m^T v^{-1}$.

In case of normality, the Student's t-test should be used. We should imagine that a normal distribution ought to be used, but in real cases, the mean and the standard deviation are only estimated through a small set of realizations. The Student's distribution takes into account the number of realizations: if this number increases, it tends to the Gaussian distribution. Figure 4.4 shows that for low numbers, the probability in the tails part is higher than for the Gaussian distribution.

Let us consider a given distribution (μ, σ) known through a set of n realizations and T the result of a test $(T = \mu/(\sigma/\sqrt{n}))$. The cumulative distribution function will be lower for a lower n. In other terms, and as an application to statistical tests, the value of the testing variable T should be higher to reach 95% confidence if the number of realizations n is lower. The less information we have on the result (here n), the greater the difference between the two situations should be (compared to the experimental standard deviation) in order to reach a conclusion.

In practice, the Student's t-test consists of writing the testing variable T and comparing it to the threshold value T_{lim} that depends on the probability level (usually 95%), the number of realizations (in fact the number of statistical degree of freedom $\nu = n - 1$) and the questions: do you want to see a difference between two quantities A and B? (in which case the test is bilateral); or do you want to see that quantity A is higher/lower than quantity B? (in which case the test is unilateral). A bilateral test means that the threshold value would be 97.5% or 2.5% to reach 95% probability to show $A \neq B$. A unilateral test means that the threshold value would be 95% (for $A > B$) or 5% (for $A < B$).

The Mann–Whitney test allows for the comparison of two means not following a normal distribution, the tests of each group being independent. The Wilkoxon test is designed for paired test and compares the average difference to zero. The principle is the same for these two tests: regardless of the statistical law of the two groups, the probability that a random term in the first group is greater than a random term in the second group is 0.5 if their means are equal[1]. It is therefore necessary to examine all possible comparisons between the elements of each group and establish two scores, by comparing the first group with the second (U_{xy}), then by comparing the second with the first group (U_{yx}). In the first case, each time an element of the first group is greater than an element of the second, the U_{xy} score increases by 1. If an element of the first group has an identical value to an element of the second, the U_{xy} score increases by 0.5. The same goes for the second case for U_{yx}. The sum of the two scores is equal to the number of possible combinations, that is, the product of the number of tests of each group $n_1 \times n_2$. It is then sufficient to check that the value of the smaller of the two scores is less than a tabulated value. Tables for Wilkoxon and Mann–Whitney are different, since the Wilkoxon test is based on a single group.

If the numbers of tests n_1 and n_2 are greater than 10, the variable of U approximately follows a normal distribution of variance.

1 In the case of the Wilkoxon test, the second group is identically zero.

$$\sigma_u^2 = n_1 \times n_2 \times (n_1 + n_2)/12 \qquad [8.2]$$

It is then sufficient to center and reduce the U statistic and use in a parametric test with a normal distribution.

The *t*-test and *U*-test aim to give the same information. *U*-test can be used in more diverse situations than the *t*-test, as there is no assumption on the distribution. Unfortunately, the *U*-test is also less sensitive than the *t*-test. For that reason, the *t*-test must be preferred when it is applicable.

8.3.4. *Example: pressure applied by a compression bandage*

Methodology	Stretch	U_{AB}	U_{BA}
B	1.282	6	0
A	1.288	0	5
B	1.288	5	0
B	1.29	5	0
A	1.294	0	3
B	1.294	4	0
A	1.298	0	2
B	1.308	3	0
A	1.312	0	1
B	1.313	2	0
A	1.321	0	0
A	1.325	0	0
		$U_{AB} = 25$	$U_{BA} = 11$

Table 8.2. *Mann–Whitney test for venous compression therapy. Results are presented in decreasing order*

Different compression stocking application methodologies are used in the treatment of venous insufficiency. According to the first method, denoted as methodology A, the average deformation of the band is $m_1 = 1.28$ ($s_1^2 = 2.5 \times 10^{-3}$, $n_1 = 15$). According to the second method, denoted as methodology B, the deformation is $m_2 = 1.27$ ($s_2^2 = 2.5 \times 10^{-3}$, $n_1 = 15$). However, in this case, the Shapiro–Wilk test invalidates the assumption of normality. It is therefore necessary to use a nonparametric test. The obtained values are summarized in Table 8.2. In this case, $U_{BA} > 8$, which means that the hypothesis cannot be rejected. With this information at our disposal, it is impossible to conclude that the effects of two application methodologies are statistically different.

8.4. Linear regression

8.4.1. *Mathematics of linear regression*

Linear regression is a simple way to build an experimental model using a set of data. It requires us to identify a response Y that depends on a set of factors x_i (e.g. age, BMI and dose). Generally speaking, the experimentalist disposes of n experiments (therefore n equations) to identify the values of $m + 1$ linear coefficients and possibly $C_m^2 = m!/\{(m-2)!\,2!\}$ first-order interactions. To the extent that there are more experiments than variables, the problem is one of minimization. Each of the n achievements can be written particularly in the form of a linear experimental model, as presented in relationships [8.3], [8.4] or [8.5].

$$f(x) = \beta_0 + \sum_{i=1}^{m} \beta_i x_i \qquad [8.3]$$

$$\forall x \in E, f(x) = \beta_0 + \sum_{i=1}^{m} \beta_i x_i + \sum\sum_{i<j} \beta_{ij} x_i x_j \qquad [8.4]$$

$$\forall x \in E, f(x) = \beta_0 + \sum_{i=1}^{m} \beta_i x_i + \sum_{i=1} \beta_{ii}\, x_i^2 + \sum\sum_{i<j} \beta_{ij} x_i\, x_j \qquad [8.5]$$

All of the relationships corresponding to the n realizations can be synthesized in a standard way in the matrix form [8.6]:

$$\vec{Y} = X\vec{\beta} + \vec{\epsilon} \quad [8.6]$$

In equation [8.6], $\vec{Y}$ is the vector of the realizations, $\boldsymbol{X}$ is the matrix of the experimental model, containing all of the experimental conditions, and $\vec{\beta}$ is the vector of the model parameters. The term $\vec{\epsilon}$ sums up the errors (experimental and model adjustment error) that we try to minimize, thanks to the writing of the functional:

$$\begin{aligned} J(\vec{\beta}) &= \frac{1}{2}\| X\vec{\beta} - \vec{Y}\|^2 \\ &= \frac{1}{2}\,{}^t(X\vec{\beta} - \vec{Y})(X\vec{\beta} - \vec{Y}) \end{aligned} \quad [8.7]$$

The search for an extremum of $J(\vec{\beta})$ is performed by deriving the functional with respect to the different variables β_i, $i \in \mathbb{N}$. If we note that $\hat{\vec{\beta}}$ is the approximate solution minimizing the least-squares deviations, the mathematical expression is given as:

$$\nabla_\beta J(\hat{\vec{\beta}}) = 0 \Leftrightarrow {}^t X(X\hat{\vec{\beta}} - \vec{Y}) = 0 \quad [8.8]$$

By expanding equation [8.8], if the expression $({}^tXX)$ is invertible, that is, if the number of independent experiments is greater than that of the unknowns and if the conditioning of this matrix is correct, the approximate solution in the least square sense is given as:

$$\hat{\vec{\beta}} = ({}^tXX)^{-1}\,{}^tX\vec{Y} \quad [8.9]$$

Therefore, it is possible to estimate the quantity of interest $\hat{\vec{Y}}$ noted by using relationship [8.6].

$$\hat{\vec{Y}} = X({}^tXX)^{-1}\,{}^tX\vec{Y} \quad [8.10]$$

The covariance matrix for $\hat{\vec{\beta}}$ is written as:

$$\text{Var}(\hat{\vec{\beta}}) = [({}^t XX)^{-1}\,{}^t X]\,\text{Var}(\vec{Y})\,{}^t[({}^t XX)^{-1}\,{}^t X] \qquad [8.11]$$

Under the assumption that the variance on $\vec{Y}$ is constant over time and value (homoscedasticity), variances on $\hat{\vec{\beta}}$ and $\hat{\vec{Y}}$ are given as:

$$\text{Var}(\hat{\vec{\beta}}) = \sigma_Y^2\,({}^t XX)^{-1} \qquad [8.12]$$

$$\text{Var}(\hat{\vec{Y}}) = \sigma_Y^2[X({}^t XX)^{-1}\,{}^t X] \qquad [8.13]$$

Even if it is almost impossible in usual clinical trials, the linear regression would be better if the matrix $({}^t XX)$ was well conditioned, meaning that the global error is minimized (the determinant is close to 1) or that the error is the same at every point taken at the same distance from the center on the experimental domain ($X({}^t XX)^{-1}\,{}^t X$ is diagonal and the diagonal term is constant).

8.4.2. *Analysis of variance*

In the context of high variability, the model quality must be checked. To what extent does this model fit the data? Is it possible to classify the effects and decide the influence of a given parameter on the result? Using the linear regression can also be necessary for hypothesis testing, to remove confounding effects or to test global effect.

ANOVA is a method that could answer these questions, commonly used in clinical trials. It consists of comparing the amplitudes of variation obtained experimentally and with the linear regression model. The sum of square total (SST) and the sum of square of the regression (SSR) are defined as:

$$\text{SST} = \sum_{i=1}^{n}(Y_i - \bar{Y})^2 \qquad [8.14]$$

$$\text{SSR} = \sum_{i=1}^{n}(\hat{Y} - \bar{Y})^2 \qquad [8.15]$$

SST measures the total variance of the experimental results, and SSR measures the total variance of the regression model. The difference between the two shows the discrepancy between the experiment and the model. The sum of square error (SSE) is written as:

$$\text{SSE} = \text{SST} - \text{SSR} = \sum_{i=1}^{n}(Y_i - \hat{Y}_i)^2 \qquad [8.16]$$

But this error may be due to the bias related to the lack of fit of the model or to dispersion related to the experimental variability. By assuming that the dispersion of measurements is constant over time and for different operating conditions, and by defining n^* as the number of different experimental conditions, it is possible to determine the indicators of lack of fit (SSLOF) and pure error (SSPE):

$$SSLOF = \sum_{i=1}^{n^*}(\hat{Y}_i - \bar{Y}_i)^2 \qquad [8.17]$$

$$SSPE = \sum_{i=1}^{n^*}\sum_{u=1}^{c_i}(Y_i^{(u)} - \bar{Y}_i)^2 \qquad [8.18]$$

In these definitions, $\hat{Y}_i$ is the best estimate for Y in the sense of the least square fit, $\bar{Y}_i$ is the mean value of experimental results and $Y_i^{(u)}$ is the uth realization for the ith experimental condition.

However, the sums of squares SST, SSR, SSLOF and SSPE automatically increase with the number of measurement points. To allow for comparison between models of different complexity, obtained for a different number of points (patients here), these indicators must be averaged, dividing them by the number of degrees of statistical freedom associated with them. We achieve as follows (with n: number of tests; n^*: number of experimental conditions; and p: number of parameters):

$$MSR = \frac{SSR}{p-1} \quad [8.19]$$

$$MSE = \frac{SSE}{n-p} \quad [8.20]$$

$$MSLOF = \frac{SSLOF}{n^*-p} \quad [8.21]$$

$$MSPE = \frac{SSPE}{n-n^*} \quad [8.22]$$

Equation [8.20] clearly shows that an estimate of the error makes no sense if the number of tests is equal to the number of parameters. Similarly, there is no possibility of estimating the lack of fit if the number of experimental conditions corresponds to the number of parameters [8.21] or of estimating the pure error if there is no repetition of at least one experimental condition [8.22].

These quantities can be used to calculate the famous – but not so well known – coefficient of determination R^2. However, R^2 tends to increase mechanically with the number of variables in a model. It is therefore not suitable for comparing models with a different number of variables. In this case, it is preferable to use the adjusted coefficient of determination, corrected for degrees of freedom.

$$R^2 = \frac{SSR}{SST} = 1 - \frac{SSE}{SST} \quad [8.23]$$

$$R^2_{aj} = 1 - \frac{(1-R^2)(n-1)}{n-p-1} \quad [8.24]$$

In general terms, some tests arise from linear regression (Table 8.3). In order to check the model validity, that is, the extent to which the parameters of the model explain the variance, a test compares the mean square regression and the mean square error. If the value is high, then most of the variance is in the model. Since the test is based on the ratio of two variances (following a X^2 distribution), it follows the Fisher–Snedecor distribution (F-distribution). But even if the main part of the variance is in the model, this does not detail how the model works. A second global way to test the model is to compare the error that should be related to the lack of fit and that of the pure error. Again, this is a ratio between two variances, and it follows an F-distribution. Lastly, to estimate the significativity of the β_i parameters of the model, the usual test compares the estimate value $\hat{\vec{\beta}}$ to its variance. The distribution is that of $\hat{\vec{\beta}}$ that should be a normal distribution, so the effective test is the Student's *t*-test.

Question	Test	Statistic law
Model validity	$t = \frac{MSR}{MSE}$	Fisher–Snedecor (F)
Model adjustment	$T = \frac{MSLOF}{MSPE}$	Fisher–Snedecor (F)
Parameter β_i significativity	$t = \frac{\hat{\beta}}{\sqrt{Var(\hat{\beta})}}$	Student's test (t)

Table 8.3. *Statistical tests for linear regression*

In the medical field, if the regression is made for a single factor (e.g. three groups of ages), the test assessing the model validity is called *one-way* ANOVA. There is no information on each value for this factor. The post hoc test can discriminate if the groups are statistically different, but the probability of having an error at least once among comparisons increases rapidly: $1-(1-\alpha)^C$. The usual way then is to adjust the acceptance level for each group. The most classical one is the Bonferroni correction, where each of the p parameters is tested with a confidence level α/p, where α is the global acceptance level[2].

The simultaneous study of two factors is called "two-way ANOVA"; more generally, the study of multiple factors (dependent variables) is called "multivariate analysis of variance" (MANOVA).

8.4.3. *Correlation between parameters*

If the objective is only to find some correlation between parameters, a linear regression analysis is not necessary and classically, the Pearson correlation coefficient is calculated. Even if it is not explicit, the Pearson correlation is based on a linear assumption. It is written as:

$$\rho_{X,Y} = \frac{cov(X,Y)}{\sigma_x \sigma_y} \quad [8.25]$$

$\rho_{X,Y}$	**Interpretation**
0.7 or higher	Very strong positive relationship
0.4–0.7	Strong positive relationship
0.3–0.4	Moderate positive relationship
0.2–0.3	Weak positive relationship
0.1–0.2	No or negligible relationship
0	Theoretical zero correlation
–0.1 to –0.2	No or negligible relationship
–0.2 to –0.3	Weak negative relationship
–0.3 to –0.4	Moderate negative relationship
–0.4 to –0.7	Strong negative relationship
–0.7 or lower	Very strong negative relationship

Table 8.4. *Statistical tests for linear regression*

2 In many references, this acceptance level is called the p-value and is usually set to 0.05. Here, this naming is not used to avoid confusion with the number of parameters usually called p in ANOVA references: https://statisticsbyjim.com/anova/post-hoc-tests-anova/.

The correlation coefficient can be negative or positive. In fact, there is no correlation if $\rho_{X,Y} = 0$. Y increases with X if $\rho_{X,Y} \geq 0$ and decreases with X if $\rho_{X,Y} \leq 0$. A direct interpretation of $\rho_{X,Y}$ is often given with the following limits.

Statistics for the correlation coefficient to be different from zero must be written. The random variable t follows a Student's distribution:

$$t = \frac{|\rho_{X,Y}|}{\sqrt{(\frac{1-\rho_{X,Y}^2}{n-2})}} \quad [8.26]$$

Again, statistics is a whole world, and it is possible to find more tests, for example, Spearman's rank correlation coefficient and Kendall's rank correlation coefficient, which are based on ranks, without normality assumption.

PERSONAL PRACTICE.– A famous historical saying is continually attributed to King Henry III of France. About the body of the Duke of Guise lying at his feet, the king is said to have exclaimed: "he is taller dead than alive!". Does a person measure the same height lying down and standing up?

1) From the collected data (see extra material online in Molimard (2023)) and the general methodology described above, check if this statement is true. JASP software can be used[3].

2) Bonus question: Are women the same height as men?

PERSONAL PRACTICE.– During a study on knee braces, the level of skin deformation in the vicinity of the brace is sought. Eleven trials are performed on healthy subjects aged 20–27 years old, with five men and six women.

3 Available at: https://jasp-stats.org/download/.

Additional data were collected, such as skin fold and BMI (see extra material online in Molimard (2023)).

1) Do male and female populations have the same characteristics in terms of BMI/age/cutaneous ply thickness/strain? Be careful with the test used.

2) Do strain and cutaneous ply thickness correlate? First visualize the correlation plot, then perform the appropriate test.

3) In order to go further, a linear regression is performed with strain as a function of other variables. What are the statistically relevant factors?

9

Longitudinal Practice with Sensor Design

This practice is built in four steps and a defense. Students will gather in groups of three to six and follow the logical steps from ideation to signal processing.

9.1. Design

A one-page report is expected at the end of the session.

Sleep apnea is a common sleep disorder, with 10% prevalence (30% of the elderly). It is related to a degraded quality of life (daytime sleepiness, impaired alertness); however, the consequences to health could not be more important, with increased risk of cardiovascular problems.

We propose here to follow the breathing regularity with a small inertial measurement unit (IMU) placed on the chest delivering information to a computer (smartphone) wireless through the Bluetooth protocol. Prototyping can be done easily with Arduino-like boards.

1) Find information on sleep apnea. How is the diagnosis made, and how is the disease monitored and controlled?

2) What is the rough information given by the IMU? Imagine the derived information that could be relevant in the context of sleep apnea.

3) It is important to have a state of the art patent review to define a patenting strategy for this new device. Go to open-source patent repositories[1] to detect concurrent ideas and propose a strategy.

In the first step, more in the academic context of a longitudinal practice, open-source repositories are enough, but this should be completed with more systematic resources.

4) Then, we will clarify the advantages and drawbacks of this solution. In order to justify this choice, you should answer the following questions:

– Compare Bluetooth communication to other transmission protocols.

– What incidence would the choice of an SD card have on the user's experience?

– What data management would you imagine? In particular, to whom should the data be sent?

9.2. Session 2: building an IMU-based sensor

A one-page report is expected at the end of the session.

We propose the following set-up:

– an Arduino board (e.g. Teensy 3.2, PJRC, Sherwood, Oregon, USA);

1 Available at: http://www.freepatentsonline.com/; http://www.google.com/patents; https://www.lens.org/.

– a three-axis accelerometer/three-axis gyroscope IMU (e.g. Sparkfun MPU6050);

– a Bluetooth HC06 board;

– a power bank;

– cables.

9.2.1. *Step 1: software installation*

– Install the last Arduino IDE with appropriate board and IMU library (e.g. MPU6050) on a personal computer. Verify the communication with the board by uploading a simple program (e.g. blink) (Arduino IDE is freely available at https://www.arduino.cc/, with tutorials and examples).

– Install your favorite scientific computing software (e.g. GNU Octave; Eaton et al. 2023) on a personal computer with the appropriate signal processing toolbox. Octave is a free GNU software that can be found at https://www.gnu.org/software/octave/download.html and a free package list is given at https://gnu-octave.github.io/packages/ and can be installed using the command pkg install forge package_name. Signal and statistics toolboxes ought to be installed. Many lectures on Octave are available online[2].

– Install Serial Bluetooth terminal application on a smartphone.

9.2.2. *Step 2: wiring*

We need to carefully wire the bluetooth device and the IMU to our board. Basically, for each element, two wires are

2 For example: Jason Lachnie, *Introduction to GNU Octave – A brief tutorial for linear algebra and calculus students*: http://www.wcc.vccs.edu/sites/default/files/Introduction-to-GNU-Octave.pdf.

used for the power supply and two wires for the communication. It is mandatory here to refer to the specific set-up. Figure 9.1 reproduces the wiring used to validate the practice.

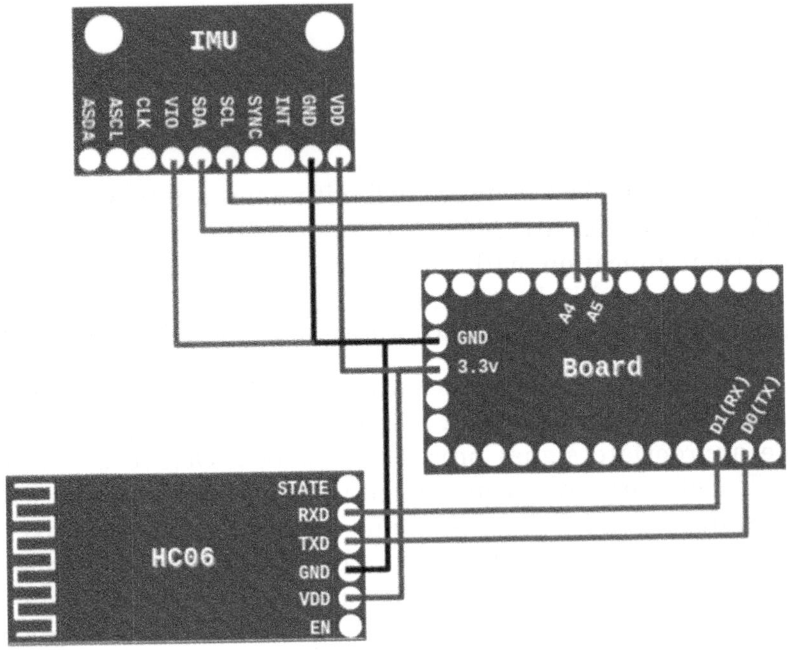

Figure 9.1. *Wiring the Arduino-compatible board to Bluetooth and IMU devices. Note that IMU needs a clear addressing by setting VIO input to 0 or 3.3 V. For a color version of this figure, see www.iste.co.uk/molimard/biomedicaldevices.zip*

9.2.3. *Step 3: uploading code to the board*

An example of code is given in Molimard (2023). Now, open the microcontroller program MPU6050Madwick.ino and upload it to the system. After an initialization loop, the device starts emitting. It can be powered either by the computer, a LiPO battery or a power bank.

To verify the signal emission, the simplest way is to use a serial Bluetooth terminal application on a smartphone, even if solutions exist on computers. Firstly, pair the smartphone with the Bluetooth HC06 (there should be a password, 000 or 123 in most cases).

9.3. Session 3: signal procession and metrology

A one-page report is expected at the end of the session

Now it is time to use the sensors. Before going to signal processing for a given experiment, it is important to qualify the sensor metrology.

The protocol for signal transmission of the data is the following:

1) Record the first result on the smartphone and transmit the data to the computer through a shared library or email.

2) Open the values under Octave (data-tabulated values can be read using dlmread with option "\t").

3) Time is in the first column, then accelerations (in x, y and z) and rotation speed (in x, y and z). Carefully read the data and try to physically understand the results.

The first step when setting up a sensor is a metrological verification. This task may become difficult in the case of time-dependent data, as in the case of acceleration or rotation speed. Some simple tests can be done anyway.

– Record data for 30 s using the sensor kept fixed on the table. Then import data under Octave.

- What is the actual sampling frequency? How variable is it (you may use a boxplot representation here)?

- Is there any long-term variation of recorded data? You can use the polyfit function first, and then write a statistical test to determine if the drift is statistically different from zero.

- After removing eventual drift, quantify the sensor resolution in each direction.

– Record data over 30 s by moving the sensor in any spatial orientation and any direction. Then import data under Octave.

- Is the sensor sensitivity dependent on the orientation? You can calculate the acceleration amplitude along with time.

9.4. Session 4: sleep apnea

This last session will explore basic signal processing to detect sleep abnormalities. Chest movement is periodic and sleep apnea can be seen as the detection of any deviation from usual in a periodic signal (amplitude or frequency).

– Explore the signal processing toolbox in Octave and decide what kind of transformation should represent better the signal and outline any deviation. You might think of:

- Fourier transform: *y* = ***fft****(x,n).*

- Short-term Fourier transform: *y* = **stft** *(x, win_size).*

- *Spectogram: S = specgram(x).*

– Simulate a 5 min calm breathing. Reproduce the same test with some perturbation by blocking the volunteer's nostrils for a few seconds.

– Examine the capacity of each representation in detecting the events, while not giving false positives.

– Perform the same test on volunteers in the classroom.

- Extract the data from IMU sensor for each patient.

- Quantify the number of events for each patient.

- Show the confusion matrix in the defined conditions.

- Draw the true positive rate versus false positive rate using a receiver operating characteristic (ROC) curve, and estimate the classifier quality using the area under the curve (AUC).

Perform the same test on volunteers in the classroom.

10

Longitudinal Practice Focused on Clinical Trial

This chapter is divided into four steps and a defense. Students will gather in groups of three to six and follow the logical steps from ideation to pre-statistical analysis. The objective is to write a convincing clinical trial file and to defend it in front of an institutional review board. A complete clinical trial form is given in the Appendix. Not all sections need to be completed in the academic context, but we encourage students to read all the documents and make links with the ethics and quality concerns developed in Chapter 6.

10.1. Session 1: frailty problems

The population is getting older in industrialized countries, first in Europe and in Japan, but very soon in China and the United States. This results in a lot of challenges for the social organization and healthcare systems. Frailty is one of these. Frailty is "theoretically defined as a clinically recognizable state of increased vulnerability resulting from aging-associated decline in reserve and function across multiple physiologic systems such that the ability to cope with everyday or acute stressors is compromised" (Fried et al. 2001; Xue 2011).

1) Find a more practical definition of frailty, based on medical practice for its diagnosis.

2) What are the main protocols to evaluate the frailty level of a patient?

3) Who are the different people involved in the care of the syndrome?

4) Frailty is a multi-form syndrome, and so far a complete answer from the engineering point view might be strictly out of reach. Exchange with your neighbors on the various ways (mention at least three) to help patients and physicians to evaluate or mitigate frailty.

5) What is the incidence of frailty in the patient's life? What is the prevalence and the healthcare cost associated with it?

This session should give most of the medical background (section C.4. in the Appendix).

10.2. Session 2: project draft

Each group proposes a solution (physical device, software or application, etc.) to address a health problem related to frailty.

Product ideation can follow the path described in "Medical Device Innovation Handbook"[1], but without giving too much importance to the commercial viability (patenting, market, etc.) and it should be original. It is also possible to re-use an existing project. The effort must be put into the relevance of the clinical trial.

1 Available at: https://sites.google.com/a/umn.edu/mdih/.

This session should help in writing the medical device description (section C.3. in the Appendix).

10.3. Session 3: design of a clinical trial (1)

Before going into technical (statistical) details, it is important to define the primary and secondary research questions.

The questions must be put into perspective with the state of the art in the scientific literature. PubMed[2] is the reference scientific database. Lens[3] and Google Scholar[4] are more general but can help with wider free access content.

The scientific justification should become an extensive work. Here, please make it simple and stay reasonable in your research. Firstly, identify the right keywords for your research and extract 5–10 papers. It then becomes possible to construct the scientific justification on the abstracts.

This session should help in writing sections C.5, C.6 and C.7 in the Appendix.

10.4. Session 4: design of a clinical trial (2)

This session will go through the usual questions of a clinical trial, for example, level of risk and number of participants.

Most of the questions are very quick to answer and justification should be given only in specific cases (e.g. trial on vulnerable people). It is worth reading them as it goes over most of the ethics issues.

---

2 Available at: https://www.ncbi.nlm.nih.gov/pmc/.

3 Available at: https://www.lens.org/.

4 Available at: https://scholar.google.fr/.

The trickiest part is the number of participants. A lot of professionals are still not comfortable with this issue. Usually, people use previous studies to quantify their cohort. In any case, it derives from the statistical test related to the primary question; and by knowing the expected dispersion and the level of the effect, it is possible to calculate the number of participants (e.g. https://biostatgv.sentiweb.fr/).

This session should help in writing sections C.8–C.13 and D, E and F in the Appendix.

10.5. Session 5: defense in front of the IRB

The defense will be a 15-min defense and questions for each group.

Appendix

Clinical Trial Form

Application for a Recognized Research Ethics Committee (REC) Opinion on a Clinical Trial on a Medicinal Product for Human Use.[1]

This application form should be completed and submitted by the chief investigator (the person who takes primary responsibility for the conduct of the clinical trial). It should be filled out in language comprehensible to a layperson.

TRIAL IDENTIFICATION

A.1.
EudraCT No.
Title of clinical trial
Submission date

1 This document derives from the "2012 Guidance on the Application for Recognised Ethics Committee Opinion and the ethical review of clinical trials on medicinal products for human use" (see: https://assets.gov.ie/54581/5a0db66907fb473a9c5d9698b691528f.pdf). Note that it is a general purpose clinical trial form, closely fitting with ethics considerations. For dedicated forms for medical devices, the reader should visit: https://health.ec.europa.eu/document/download/13265ec7-1776-41af-afb6-e0a64bc407b5_en?filename=mdcg_2021-8_en.pdf.

A.2.	
Proposed start date (first person first visit)	dd/mm/yyyy
Proposed end date (last person last visit)	dd/mm/yyyy
Expected duration (years/months)	dd/mm/yyyy

APPLICANT IDENTIFICATION

B.1. Chief investigator
Name: Title: Position: Qualifications: Address: Tel: Fax: E-mail: (***Please submit a 2-page CV for the chief investigator***)[2]

B.2. Sponsor
(Not detailed for this exercise)

2 Some lines are left gray: please do not fill in: they are given for information only.

DETAILS OF THE CLINICAL TRIAL

C.1.	
Has this or a similar application been previously submitted for review to this or any other ethics committee in the country? If yes, please give details.	Yes No

C.2. Multi-center clinical trials	
Is this trial a multi-center trial? If yes, please submit a list of all proposed sites in the country and proposed investigators including contact no./e-mail.	Yes No

Does this trial involve third countries?	Yes No
Have you received permission from each of the above sites in the country to conduct this trial?	Yes No

C.3. Substance/medical device	
Name of the substance/medical device, which you propose to administer during the clinical trial. Description of the substance/medical device. Typical length: 10 lines + 1 figure	

(Somatic cell therapy and gene therapy or genetically modified cells sections have been removed for document compactness.)

C.4. Motivation/medical background

Please specify here what is the medical background justifying a new clinical approach.

This section aims at clarifying the importance of the problem and the expected progress for the society.

Typical length: 1/2–1 page

C.5. Primary research question/objective

Please specify the primary research question/objective.

The primary question should be answered with statistics tools; the trial is build to warranty a statistically funded result.

Typical length: 1–5 lines

C.6. Secondary research question/objective

Please specify the secondary research question/objective.

Typical length: 1–5 lines

C.7. Scientific justification

What is the scientific justification for the clinical trial?

Scientific justification gives a state of the art on the subject and extracts the scientific question.

Typical length: 1/2–1 page

C.8. Methods and design of the clinical trial

Give a brief description of the methods and design of the proposed clinical trial, e.g. randomized and controlled. This should also include details of the duration of research participant involvement and exactly what procedures they will undergo.

A detailed description is required here. It should describe how the quality of the test is maximized and how the drawbacks for the patients are minimized.

Typical length: 1–2 pages

C.9.

Will treatment be withheld from research participants as a result of taking part in the clinical trial?	Yes No

If yes, please give details.

C.10. Adverse effects

What are the potential adverse effects, risks or hazards for research participants either from giving or withholding medications, devices, ionizing radiation, or from other interventions, which may cause inconvenience or changes to lifestyle?

C.12. Benefits

What are the potential benefits for research participants?

C.13. Research participant follow-up

What procedures are in place to monitor the health of the research participants during the trial or when they are no longer involved in the trial?

DETAILS OF TRIAL PARTICIPANTS

D.1. Number of participants

How many research participants and controls are expected to participate at each site in Ireland?

Give any statistical justification for this choice.

D.2. Recruitment

How will research participants/controls be identified and recruited?

D.3. Inclusion criteria

What are the inclusion criteria?

D.4. Exclusion criteria

What are the exclusion criteria?

D.5. Patient withdrawing

What criteria exist for withdrawing research participants prematurely?

What is the procedure for patients voluntarily withdrawing from the trial?

D.6. Vulnerable patients	
Will the participants be from any of the following groups? *(tick as appropriate)*	
Children under 16	Adults with learning disabilities
Adults who are unconscious	Adults who have a terminal illness
Adults in emergency situations	Adults with mental illness
Pregnant women/women of child-bearing age	Prisoners
Adults suffering from dementia	Healthy volunteers
Those who could be considered to be vulnerable or have a particularly dependent relationship with the investigator, for example, those in care homes and medical students.	
Please justify their inclusion, outlining how the trial is expected to benefit research participants.	

(NOTE: Parts 4 and 5 of Schedule 1 of the European Communities (Clinical Trials on Medicinal Products for Human Use) Regulations 2004 clearly outline the conditions and principles, which apply in relation to the treatment of Minors or Incapacitated Adults who are participants in medical research.)

D.7.	
Will research participants be reimbursed for expenses?	Yes No
If yes, please clarify.	

D.8.	
Will they receive any incentives for taking part in the clinical trial? If yes, please clarify.	Yes No

D.9.	
Will the participant's general practitioner be notified of his or her participation in the trial? If no, please clarify.	Yes No

Informed consent

E.1.	
Will written informed consent be obtained? If yes, who will be responsible for obtaining (qualifications and experience)? If no, please justify.	Yes No

E.2.
Give details of the manner in which consent will be obtained. Please attach copies of both the information leaflet and consent form.

E.3.	
What arrangements have been made for research participants who might not adequately understand verbal or written information?	

Confidentiality[3]

F.1.	
Does the proposed clinical trial involve the retention of biological material (tissue, bodily fluids) or data derived from them? If yes, for what period of time will the biological material and/or data be retained?	Yes No

F.2.
How will data security be maintained?

F.3.
Who will have access to the biological material and/or data?

3 In France, this section is treated in a specific manner with a seperate CNIL declaration.

F.4.
If biological material and/or data are to be disposed of, please explain how and by whom this will be done?

F.5.
How will the results of the clinical trial be reported and disseminated (e.g. peer-reviewed journal and research participants)?

Financial arrangements

G.1.
What arrangements have been made for compensation in the event of a claim made by or on behalf of a participant?

G.2.	
Is indemnity in place for the conduct of this clinical trial? If yes, please submit a copy to the REC.	Yes No

G.3.	
Has funding for the clinical trial been secured?	Yes No
If yes, give details of funding organization(s) and amount secured and duration: Organization: Contact name: Address: Tel: Fax: E-mail: Amount:	
If no, what arrangements have been made to cover the cost of the research?	

G.4.	
Does the chief investigator or any of the investigators have any direct/indirect involvement in the outcome of the clinical trial that could in anyway be regarded as a possible conflict of interest? If yes, please explain.	Yes No

Declaration of the chief investigator

This declaration must be signed and sent to the REC together with the requisite fee before the application will be considered as valid.

– I certify that the information in this form is accurate to the best of my knowledge and I take full responsibility for it.

– I undertake to abide by the ethical principles outlined in the Declaration of Helsinki, and my obligations as set out in the International Conference on Harmonisation's Good Clinical Practice Guidelines (ICH GCP) and the European Communities (Clinical Trials on Medicinal Products for Human Use) Regulations, 2004 (S.I. No 190 of 2004).

– If the clinical trial is approved, I undertake to adhere to the study protocol and to comply with any conditions set out in the letter of approval sent by the recognized ethics committee.

– I am aware of my responsibility to be up to date and comply with the requirements of the law relating to security and confidentiality of patient or other personal data.

Signature:

Print Name:

Date: (dd/mm/yyyy)

References

ANSM (2017). Investigations cliniques de dispositifs médicaux relevant du règlement européen No. 2017/745. Partie I : Dispositions générales, DOC032 v01. ANSM [Online]. Available at: https://ansm.sante.fr/vos-demarches/industriel/demander-une-autorisation-pour-un-essai-clinique-pour-des-dispositifs-medicaux-categorie-1.

ASME (2018). Assessing credibility of computational modeling through verification and validation: Application to medical devices. ASME V&V40 [Online]. Available at: https://www.asme.org/codesstandards/find-codes-standards/assessing-credibility-ofcomputational-modeling-throughverification-and-validation application-to-medical-devices.

Audry, A. and Ghislain, J.C. (2009). *Le dispositif médical*. Presses Universitaires de France, Paris.

Bernard, C. (1856). *Introduction à l'étude de la médecine expérimentale*. Éditions Flammarion, Champs.

BIPM (2008). Evaluation of measurement data – Guide to the expression of in measurement (GUM). Document, JCGM 100:2008, Bureau International des Poids et Mesures, Paris [Online]. Available at: https://www.bipm.org/utils/common/documents/jcgm/JCGM_100_2008_F.pdf.

BIPM (2012). International vocabulary of metrology – Basic and general concepts and associated terms (VIM). Document, JCGM 200:2012. Bureau International des Poids et Mesures, Paris [Online]. Available at: https://www.bipm.org/utils/common/documents/jcgm/JCGM_200_2012.pdf.

Blausen Medical (2014). Medical gallery of Blausen Medical 2014. *WikiJournal of Medicine*, 1(2). doi: 10.15347/wjm/2014.010.

Bonnaire, R. (2015). Caractérisation mécanique des orthèses : application aux ceintures de soutien lombaire dans le cadre de la lombalgie. PhD Thesis, École de MINES Saint-Étienne, Saint-Étienne [Online]. Available at: https://tel.archives-ouvertes.fr/tel-01198808.

Bonnaire, R., Verhaeghe, M., Molimard, J., Calmels, P., Convert, R. (2014). Characterization of a pressure measuring system for the evaluation of medical devices. *Proceedings of the Institution of Mechanical Engineers, Part H: Journal of Engineering in Medicine*, 228, 1264–1274.

Brown, B.H., Lawford, P.V., Smallwood, R.H., Hose, D.R., Barber, D.C. (1999). *Medical Physics and Biomedical Engineering*. Taylor and Francis, New York.

Chassagne, F., Molimard, J., Convert, R., Giraux, P., Badel, P. (2018). Numerical model reduction for the prediction of interface pressure applied by compression bandages on the lower leg. *IEEE Transactions on Biomedical Engineering*, 65, 449–457.

Chèze, L. (2016). *Kinematic Analysis of Human Movement*. ISTE Ltd, London, and John Wiley & Sons, New York.

Eaton, J.W., Bateman, D., Hauberg, S., Wehbring, R. (2023). GNU Octave version 8.2.0 manual: A high-level interactive language for numerical computations [Online]. Available at: https://www.gnu.org/software/octave/doc/v8.2.0/.

E-infochip (2018). A definitive guide to medical device design and development [Online]. Available at: https://www.einfochips.com/resources/publications/a-definitive-guide-to-medical-device-design-and-development/.

Erdemir, A., Mulugeta, L., Ku, J.P., Drach, A., Horner, M., Morrison, T.M., Peng, G.C.Y., Vadigepalli, R., Lytton, W.W., Myers Jr, J.G. et al. (2020). Credible practice of modeling and simulation in healthcare: Ten rules from a multidisciplinary perspective. *J. Transl. Med.*, 18, 369. doi: 10.1186/s12967-020-02540-4.

Fried, L.P., Tangen, C.M., Walston, J., Newman, A.B., Hirsch, C., Gottdiener, J., Seeman, T., Tracy, R., Kop, W.J., Burke, G., McBurnie, M.N. (2001). Frailty in older adults: Evidence for a phenotype. *The Journal of Gerontology Series A*, 56(3), M146–M156 [Online]. Available at: https://academic.oup.com/biomedgerontology/article/56/3/M146/545770.

ICH (1995). Guideline for good clinical practice E6 (R2). EMA/CHMP/ICH/135/1995. *International Conference on Harmonisation of Technical Requirements for Registration of Pharmaceuticals for Human Use*, Committee for Human Medicinal Products [Online]. Available at: https://www.ema.europa.eu/en/documents/scientific-guideline/ich-e-6-r2-guideline-good-clinical-practice-step-5_en.pdf.

Keenan, E., Gethin, G., O'Connor, G., Flynn, L., Watterson, D. (2017). Investigating point to point emissivity variation of wounded tissue. National University of Ireland Galway Research Day [Online]. Available at: https://nuigulresearchday2017.files.wordpress.com/2017/04/nuigul-2017_paper_21.pdf.

Liu, S. (2014). Design controls. FDA [Online]. Available at: https://www.slideshare.net/aleksejssurskis1/design-control-prezent-fda.

Lurie, P. and Greco, D.B. (2005). US exceptionalism comes to research ethics. *Lancet*, 365(9465), 1117–1119. doi: 10.1016/S0140-6736(05)71856-0.

Madgwick, S., Harrison, A., Vaidyanathan, R. (2011). Estimation of IMU and MARG orientation using a gradient descent algorithm. In *2011 IEEE International Conference on Rehabilitation Robotics*, June 29—July 1. Rehab week Zurich, ETH Zurich Science City.

Marey, E.-J. (1883). La station de physiologie de Paris. *La Nature*, 535, 227.

Molimard, J. (2016). *Experimental Mechanics of Solids and Structures*. ISTE Ltd, London, and John Wiley & Sons, New York.

Molimard, J. (2023). Extra material for biomedical device and sensors book. Dataset. doi: 10.5281/zenodo.8424355.

Molimard, J., Bonnaire, R., Han, W.S., Convert, R., Calmels, P. (2019). In-silico pre-clinical trials are made possible by a new simple and comprehensive lumbar belt mechanical model based on the Law of Laplace including support deformation and adhesion effects. *PLOS ONE*, 14, e0212681.

Nichamin, L.D. (2009). Glaukos iStent trabecular micro-bypass. *Middle East Afr. J. Ophthalmol.*, 16(3), 138–140. doi: 10.4103/0974-9233.56218.

Pagnon, D., Domalain, M., Reveret, L. (2021). Pose2Sim: An end-to-end workflow for 3D markerless sports kinematics – Part 1: Robustness. *Sensors*, 21, 6530. doi: 10.3390/s21196530.

Pearson, K. (1901). On lines and planes of closest fit to systems of points in space. *Philosophical Magazine*, 2(6), 559–572.

Razali, N.M. and Wah, Y.B. (2011). Power comparisons of Shapiro-Wilk, Kolmogorov-Smirnov, Lilliefors and Anderson-Darling tests. *Journal of Statistical Modeling and Analytics*, 2(1), 21–33.

Thadewald, T. and Büning, H. (2007). Jarque–Bera test and its competitors for testing normality – A power comparison. *Journal of Applied Statistics*, 34(1), 87–105.

Thomas, D., Chancellor, D., Micklus, A., LaFever, S., Hay, M., Chaudhuri, S., Bowden, R., Lo, A.W. (2021). Clinical development success rates and contributing factors 2011–2020. Study, BIO, Informa Pharma Intelligence and QLS Advisors [Online]. Available at: https://go.bio.org/rs/490-EHZ-999/images/ClinicalDevelopmentSuccessRates2011_2020.pdf.

Wagner, F.B., Mignardot, J.B., Le Goff-Mignardo, C.G., Demesmaeker, R., Komi, S., Capogrosso, M., Rowald, A., Seanez, I., Caban, M., Pirondini, E. et al. (2018). Targeted neurotechnology restores walking in humans with spinal cord injury. *Nature*, 563, 65–71. doi: 10.1038/s41586-018-0649-2.

Xue, Q.-L. (2011). The frailty syndrome: Definition and natural history. *Clin. Geriatr. Med.*, 27(1), 1–15. doi: 10.1016/j.cger.2010.08.009.

EC regulation

European Commission (2017). Medical devices. Regulation (EU) 2017/745 [Online] Available at: https://ec.europa.eu/growth/single-market/european-standards/harmonised-standards/medical-devices_en.

European Commission Medical Device Coordination Group (2021). Clinical investigation application/notification documents [Online] Available at: https://health.ec.europa.eu/document/download/13265ec7-1776-41af-afb6-e0a64bc407b5_en?filename=mdcg_2021-8_en.pdf.

EUR-Lex (2010). Directive 2010/63/EU of the European Parliament and of the Council of 22 September 2010 on the protection of animals used for scientific purposes (Text with EEA relevance) [Online]. Available at: https://eur-lex.europa.eu/legal-content/EN/TXT/?uri=CELEX%3A02010L0063-20190626.

EUR-Lex (2017). Regulation (EU) 2017/745 of the European Parliament and of the Council of 5 April 2017 on medical devices, amending Directive 2001/83/EC, Regulation (EC) No 178/2002 and Regulation (EC) No. 1223/2009 and repealing Council Directives 90/385/EEC and 93/42/EEC (Text with EEA relevance) [Online]. Available at: https://eur-lex.europa.eu/legal-content/EN/TXT/?uri=CELEX%3A32017R0745.

Université de Lille (2019). Le marquage CE des dispositifs médicaux Université de Lille [Online]. Available at: https://rpn-pharmacie.univ-lille.fr/marquagece/co/MarquageCE_web.html.

FDA regulation

FDA (2002). General principles of software validation: Guidance for industry and FDA staff [Online]. Available at: https://www.fda.gov/regulatory-information/search-fda-guidance-documents/general-principles-software-validation.

FDA (2016). Reporting of computational modeling studies in medical device submissions: Guidance for industry and Food and Drug Administration staff [Online]. Available at: https://www.fda.gov/media/87586/download.

FDA (2024a). FDA medical device product classification [Online]. Available at: https://www.fda.gov/medical-devices/classify-your-medical-device/product-code-classification-database.

FDA (2024b). FDA clinical trial guidance document [Online]. Available at: https://www.fda.gov/science-research/clinical-trials-and-human-subject-protection/clinical-trials-guidance-documents.

Owda, A.Y. and Salmon, N.A. (2019). Variation in the electromagnetic signatures of the human skin with physical activity and hydration level of the skin. *Proc. SPIE 11164, Millimetre Wave and Terahertz Sensors and Technology XII*, 1116402. doi: 10.1117/12.2533162.

Viceconti, M., Pappalardo, F., Rodriguez, B., Horner, M., Bischoff, J., Musuamba Tshinanu, F. (2021). In silico trials: Verification, validation and uncertainty quantification of predictive models used in the regulatory evaluation of biomedical products. *Methods*, 185, 120–127. doi: 10.1016/j.ymeth.2020.01.011.

Index

A, C, D

E, F, I

L, M, N

O, P, Q

R, S, T

U, V, X

Other titles from

iSTE

in

Health Engineering and Society

2024

SARAZIN Marianne
Artificial Intelligence in Health
(Technological Prospects and Social Applications Set – Volume 7)

2023

BEYALA Laure
Digital Therapy: The New Age of Healthcare
(Technological Prospects and Social Applications Set – Volume 6)

CORROY Laurence, CHAUZAL-LARGUIER Christelle
Patients, Caregivers and Doctors: Devices, Issues and Representations
(Communication and Health Set – Volume 1)

SOMMER Pascal, DEBRET Romain
The Elasticity of Life: From Tissues to Humans

2022

ASSAILLY Jean-Pascal
Child Psychology: Developments in Knowledge and Theoretical Models
(Health and Patients Set – Volume 3)

CHAABANE Sondès, COUSEIN Etienne, WIESER Philippe
Healthcare Systems: Challenges and Opportunities

PAGANELLI Céline, CLAVIER Viviane
Information Practices and Knowledge in Health
(Health and Patients Set – Volume 5)

SALGUES Bruno, BARNOUIN Jacques
The Covid-19 Crisis: From a Question of an Epidemic to a Societal Questioning
(Health and Patients Set – Volume 4)

2021

BÉRANGER Jérôme
Societal Responsibility of Artificial Intelligence: Towards an Ethical and Eco-responsible AI
(Technological Prospects and Social Applications Set – Volume 4)

CORDELIER Benoit, GALIBERT Olivier
Digital Health Communications
(Technological Prospects and Social Applications Set – Volume 5)

NADOT Michel
Discipline of Nursing: Three-time Knowledge

2020

BARBET Jacques, FOUCQUIER Adrien, THOMAS Yves
Therapeutic Progress in Oncology: Towards a Revolution in Cancer Therapy?
(Health and Patients Set – Volume 2)

MORILLON Laurent, CLAVIER Viviane
Health Research Practices in a Digital Context
(Health Information Set – Volume 4)

PAILLIART Isabelle
New Territories in Health
(Health Information Set – Volume 3)

2019

CLAVIER Viviane, DE OLIVEIRA Jean-Philippe
Food and Health: Actor Strategies in Information and Communication
(Health Information Set – Volume 2)

PIZON Frank
Health Education and Prevention
(Health and Patients Set – Volume 1)

2018

HUARD Pierre
The Management of Chronic Diseases: Organizational Innovation and Efficiency

PAGANELLI Céline
Confidence and Legitimacy in Health Information and Communication
(Health Information Set – Volume 1)

2017

PICARD Robert
Co-design in Living Labs for Healthcare and Independent Living: Concepts, Methods and Tools

2015

BÉRANGER Jérôme
Medical Information Systems Ethics